Eduardo García Solís

BIOETHICS AND MORE

Eduardo García Solís

BIOETHICS AND MORE

ScienciaScripts

Imprint
Any brand names and product names mentioned in this book are subject to trademark, brand or patent protection and are trademarks or registered trademarks of their respective holders. The use of brand names, product names, common names, trade names, product descriptions etc. even without a particular marking in this work is in no way to be construed to mean that such names may be regarded as unrestricted in respect of trademark and brand protection legislation and could thus be used by anyone.

Cover image: www.ingimage.com

This book is a translation from the original published under ISBN 978-620-2-14059-1.

Publisher:
Sciencia Scripts
is a trademark of
Dodo Books Indian Ocean Ltd. and OmniScriptum S.R.L publishing group

120 High Road, East Finchley, London, N2 9ED, United Kingdom
Str. Armeneasca 28/1, office 1, Chisinau MD-2012, Republic of Moldova, Europe
Printed at: see last page
ISBN: 978-620-6-51680-4

BIOETHICS AND MORE

EDUARDO GARCÍA SOLÍS

Eduardo García-Solís: Surgeon. National Autonomous University of Mexico. Graduate of the Clinical Bioethics course, UNESCO/Graduate of the Ethics in Research course, UNESCO/Executive Director of the Bioethics Commission of the State of Campeche, Mexico.

FOREWORD

It is a privilege and an honor for me to introduce readers to the pages of this exciting book: "Bioethics and Something More", which Dr. Eduardo García Solís, a specialist in bioethics, invites me to write the prologue. This work encourages us to enter into an intellectual journey in search of a deeper and more meaningful understanding of bioethical issues that influence and shape our medical practice and our society as a whole, since it is the intersection of biodiversity, ethics and human reflection.

In these pages, the reader will find a comprehensive exploration of bioethics, beyond its fundamental concepts. Bioethics, as a multidisciplinary field, is constantly expanding and intertwining with issues of global relevance in health care, biomedical research, and the relationship between science and humanity. This work is not limited to classical theories and dilemmas; it goes beyond them to the constantly evolving frontiers of contemporary bioethics.

The book not only examines the ethical dilemmas we face in the medical field, but also considers broader issues related to biotechnology, genetics, artificial intelligence in health care, and the impact of globalization on health. In each of the 65 chapters, the author delves into ethical debates, offers critical analyses, and presents innovative perspectives to guide readers through the ethical challenges of our time.

Throughout these pages, you will find interesting facts that will illuminate your understanding of bioethics, such as the impact of technological advances on clinical decision-making, the ethical challenges posed by personalized medicine, and the historical chronology of milestones in bioethics that have shaped our modern ethics.

"Bioethics and Something More" does not only limit itself to raising ethical questions, but also invites deep reflection and the search for answers. It reminds us that bioethics is not a static field, but a constantly changing discipline that requires an open and curious mind.

As I conclude this foreword, I invite you to enter the pages of this book with an open mind and an inquisitive spirit. Bioethics is not just a discipline; it is a call to reflection, responsibility and the search for a balance between scientific progress and respect for human dignity. In Bioethics and Something More, you will find a valuable guide to explore the ethical complexities of medicine and biotechnology in our era.

Guillermo Fajardo Ortiz

Mexico City, October 2023

INTRODUCTION

To talk about Bioethics is to talk about life. There are several definitions of bioethics, all of them accurate, such as that of the National Bioethics Commission, "It is the branch of applied ethics that reflects, deliberates and makes regulatory and public policy approaches to regulate and resolve conflicts in social life, especially in the life sciences, as well as in medical practice and research that affect life on the planet, both now and in future generations. The Pan American Health Organization points out that bioethics should not be invoked after ethical principles have been broken and we are faced with an ethically questionable situation that must be resolved. Bioethics should be incorporated into the regular work of health professionals and policy makers so that public health policies are based on bioethical principles. If I were to define bioethics, I would say doing good for the sake of doing good. The basic principles of bioethics, autonomy, beneficence, non-maleficence, justice and others such as solidarity, empathy, values such as respect and honesty. In the following pages you will find articles on how bioethics is part of everyday life. It should be present in all of us, it is a claim of society, for a better life.

INDEX

AGENDA 2030

"We aspire to a world without poverty, hunger, disease and deprivation, where all forms of life can flourish; a world without fear and violence; a world in which literacy is universal, with equitable and widespread access to quality education at all levels, health care and social protection, and where physical, mental and social well-being is ensured; a world where we reaffirm our commitments to the human right to safe drinking water and sanitation, where there is improved hygiene and food is sufficient, safe, affordable and nutritious; a world whose human habitats are safe, resilient and sustainable and where there is universal access to affordable, reliable and sustainable energy supplies." These words served as the framework, for the 2030 Agenda, during the United Nations summit on sustainable development in New York. On September 25, 2015, more than 150 world leaders attended the UN Summit, including Mexico, in order to approve the Agenda for Sustainable Development which is a pathway to eradicate poverty, protect the planet and ensure prosperity for all without compromising resources for future generations. The final document, entitled "Transforming Our World: the 2030 Agenda, includes 17 Sustainable Development Goals that aim to end poverty, fight inequality and injustice, and address climate change with no one left behind by 2030. Bioethics plays a leading role in these goals, and it is inconceivable that these objectives could be achieved without the help of bioethics. The goals that underpin it are present such as the end of poverty; zero hunger; health and well-being; quality education; gender equality; clean water and sanitation; affordable and clean energy; decent work and economic growth; industry. Innovation and infrastructure; reduction of inequalities; sustainable cities and communities; responsible production and consumption; climate action; underwater life; life of terrestrial ecosystems; peace, justice and strong institutions; partnerships to achieve the goals. For this to be possible, bioethics is essential; it is not only legal but ethical to establish what is best for the disadvantaged population. The right to the enjoyment of the highest attainable standard of health is contemplated in the Constitution of the World Health Organization (WHO) "the enjoyment of the highest attainable standard of health is one of the fundamental rights of every human being without distinction of race, religion, political ideology or economic or social condition". To make this right a reality, countries must work to improve access to health care that is timely, acceptable, affordable and of appropriate quality and the availability of health services, as well as adequate living conditions and nutritious, health-promoting foods. All of these factors are closely related to other human rights, including the right to health.Is it possible that by 2030, these goals will be met? 11 years away,Or will the same thing happen as the Declaration of Alma Ata 2000, health for all in the year 2000, and all remain good intentions? For the achievement is necessary solidarity to ensure the equitable progress of all of us who make up this beautiful country, Mexico, a collective effort to eliminate all inequalities in health that are avoidable, unfair and remediable, to overcome them, it is important to note that these inequalities are rooted in social and environmental determinants that must be addressed, such as non-discrimination, availability, accessibility, acceptability, quality, accountability and universality. With the participation of all actors in society, in an honest and responsible manner, the 2030 Agenda will become a reality.

ANXIET

In this time of decision making it is normal for people to feel anxious. Anxiety is one of the most common mental disorders and manifests itself with increased breathing, the heart beats stronger, a feeling of fear, all this so that the muscles get more blood, the brain more oxygen, thus preparing the body to any situation. Anxiety can be beneficial because it can persuade you to be on time for work, study hard enough for an exam or discourage you from walking alone in dark streets. Experiencing anxiety is normal; a certain amount of anxiety can even be helpful. The problem is that sometimes the systems underlying our anxiety responses become dysregulated, so we overreact or react to the wrong situations. There are different types of anxiety such as generalized anxiety disorder which is characterized by a pattern of excessive worry about a variety of problems on most days for at least six months, often accompanied by physical symptoms such as muscle tension, pounding heart or dizziness. Social anxiety disorder, feeling significant anxiety in social situations or when required to perform in front of others, such as public speaking, or phobias of a particular animal, insect, object, situation that causes substantial anxiety. Constant anxiety imposes a cost to health, for example, anxiety increases levels of cortisol, the stress hormone, raising blood pressure, which contributes over time to heart problems, stroke, kidney disease and sexual dysfunction. Quality of life is also affected by fear of panic attacks, fear of rejection, and other features of anxiety disorders force people to avoid anxiety-provoking situations. This interferes with relationships, work, school and daily activities, causing people to isolate themselves, reject opportunities and forgo possible joys in life. There are effective treatments for anxiety, such as lifestyle changes, omitting caffeine, exercising regularly and avoiding medications or substances that can cause anxiety symptoms. Mind-body relationship, deep breathing, meditation, mindfulness, and techniques to relieve muscle tension and promote calmness are helpful. Psychotherapy, such as cognitive behavioral therapy that teaches people to challenge and reframe distorted or unhelpful anxious thinking, because thoughts influence feelings and actions. Drugs that will be prescribed by the practitioner according to the anxiety.

The human being has always wanted to live longer, for this it is necessary to practice healthy habits. Sometimes when we are young we think that we will not get sick, so we drink alcoholic beverages in excess, we do not take care of our diet and exercise is absent. And if you reach old age, life takes its toll and you develop diseases such as obesity, diabetes, cancer, hypertension and others. Is it worth it to cultivate healthy habits? After all, if you're going to gain an extra decade of life on this earth, you want to enjoy it! Follow these steps for a longer, healthier life. If you're approaching middle age, you can take steps to enjoy a longer, healthier life, one with less chance of becoming disabled or ending up in a nursing home: 1. Eat mostly plants, most of the time. That means fruits, vegetables, beans and lentils, nuts and seeds, and whole grains. Avoid eating fast or fried foods, sweets and sugary drinks, and red and processed meats (such as cold cuts) as much as possible. 2. Move your body every day as much as you can. Walking for 30 minutes a day (15 in the morning, 15 in the evening,) would give you the benefits. But even as little as 10 minutes of movement per week has been shown to have health benefits. 3. Do your best to reach a healthy weight. And remember, even a little weight loss, just a few pounds, is associated with real, positive health outcomes, such as a lower risk of diabetes in at-risk people. 4. never smoke, because there is no healthy amount of smoking. Quitting smoking at any time has important health benefits. It is never too late to quit smoking and enjoy a healthier life. 5. If you drink alcohol, keep in mind the recommended limits: one drink per day maximum for women, two drinks per day maximum for men. If you do at least four of the five healthy habits, you will have significant protection against developing any of these diseases: on average, about a decade longer to live.Why is that important? Chronic diseases such as diabetes, cancer, obesity, high blood pressure are associated with hospitalizations and even the need for nursing home care. Diabetes, for example, can lead to disabling conditions such as blindness, amputations and kidney failure requiring dialysis, or high blood pressure which is associated with higher salt intake and low potassium, resulting in low fruit and vegetable intake. These conditions are strongly associated with diet and lifestyle. So, if you want to reach old age in the best way, it is important that you are convinced that you must take care of your body. Let's have a good life. We all want to be healthy. Let's take care of ourselves, our children, our loved ones, let's be co-responsible in taking care of our health.

TO YOUNG PEOPLE WHO WANT TO BECOME SCIENTISTS

To be ethical, to forget the phrases of he who does not compromise does not advance, the lazy ones are the ones who succeed. Young people are the future of Campeche, of Mexico. In you we trust, be proud of your roots, your values, principles, that you breastfed at home because education is not simply to instruct, but to facilitate the formation of a person's character. We live in a world of consumerism, where principles and values are forgotten, remember the teaching of Rousseau that the only and authentic sense of our actions should be to seek, to provide dignity to the conditions of human existence.Be honest, be honest, so let me tell you a story, although this is not a story, it is a fraud on scientific integrity.In 1998, Andrew Wakefield and 12 of his colleagues published a case series in Lancet, (Wakefield A.J, Murch SH, Anthony A, et al. Ileal-lymphoid-nodular hyperplasia non-specific colitis, and pervasive devalopmental disorder in children. Lancet 1998,351:637-641). In which it was suggested that vaccination against measles, mumps and rubella may predispose to behavioral regression and pervasive developmental disorder in children. It is now 21 years later and fear of vaccination still persists in some communities, mainly in the United States and Europe. Despite the fact that it has been proven that there is no relationship between the measles, rubella and mumps MMR vaccine and autism. The study consisted of a small sample size (n = 12), the uncontrolled design and the speculative nature of the conclusions described a series of cases corresponding to eleven boys and one girl, between 3 and 10 years of age, consecutively seen in the gastroenterology unit, all of them with intestinal involvement and developmental disorders. Intestinal abnormalities ranged from lymphoid nodular hyperplasia to ulcers. Neurological disorders included autism (nine patients), post-viral or post-vaccinal encephalitis (two cases), and a disintegrative psychosis or Heller's disease. The authors' interpretation associated the intestinal and neuropsychological disturbances, and suggested the MMR vaccine as a trigger. In the original study, Wakefield stated that there were traces of measles virus in the intestinal mucosa of the 12 children tested. The paper was widely publicized, and vaccination rates began to decline because parents were concerned about the risk of autism after vaccination. Almost immediately thereafter, epidemiological studies were conducted and published, refuting the proposed link between vaccination and autism. A doctor who assisted him in that research came out to say publicly that, in fact, the virus had not been found, and that Wakefield had ignored that fact in order not to harm the study. As a result, in February 2010, the editors of The Lancet retracted Wakefield's article. The General Medical Council of the United Kingdom ruled that Wakefield was ineligible for the study.the practice of the profession, describing their behavior as irresponsible, unethical and misleading. Once such a story reaches the market, it is difficult to disprove it later. So research integrity is not just another component of the research enterprise, it is a crucial component, without integrity there is no good science, no possibility of development and no possibility of hope for viable development. This episode invites reflection on the credibility and trustworthiness of authorities and professionals to the public, as well as the misgivings that can arise when potential conflicts of interest arise between professionals, industry, journals and the public. One aspect of particular interest is that of distorted expectations about the potential of health interventions, including vaccination, especially with respect to the individual and collective dimensions of prevention. It is clear that assessments can be very disparate and that not all opinions are of equal value. Although in principle it can be assumed that the experts are more authoritative, the arguments should be given the greatest attention. Hence the responsibility of the media in echoing comments and assessments of dubious value or amplifying the fears of the population, but also that of the health authorities when they are not accountable for the consequences of their decisions and, of course, that of clinicians and health professionals both in their professional conduct and when we express our opinions in public, since our attitudes and behavior influence the public, so that we must take into account the possible consequences that can be more disorienting than anything else. Although this prudence is required for the most vulnerable groups of the population, particularly minors, and only advisable if we are dealing with adult citizens, who are supposed to be mature and responsible. In any case, as it will be the citizens who will suffer or enjoy the consequences, depending on the case, it is the duty of all citizens to empower themselves, which requires accurate information and judgment, but above all will. Scientists who publish their research have the ethical responsibility to ensure the highest standards of research design, data collection, data analysis, data reporting and interpretation of findings; there can be no compromises because any error, any deception, can cause harm to patients and damage to the cause of science. Let's remember that, according to WHO, vaccines today save between 2 and 3 million lives a year worldwide.After reading these lines, you will agree that integrity is fundamental in daily life as well as in the profession we desire.

References

• Litewka, S. The impact of fraud in scientific research. The disclosure of bioethics, 2013, Secretaria de Salud/Comisión Nacional de Bioética.

• A. Segura Benedicto, The putative association between MMR vaccine and autism and vaccination refusal Gac Sanit. 2012;26(4):366-371 – La MMR vaccine and autism: sensation, refutation, retraction and fraud. TS Sathyanarayana Raoy Chittaranjan Andrade

• MMR vaccine and autism: sensation, refutation, retraction, and fraud. Indian J Psychiatry . 2011April-June; 53 (2): 95-96.

TO THE CHILDREN

What are the prolongation of existence?

Love your parents, grandparents, siblings, cousins, aunts and uncles, family. Nothing is more important than family. Have friends, friendship is a precious commodity. Do good to everyone. Help those who have less and do not expect a reward. Take care of your pets, they depend on you, they are your responsibility. When studying, always try to be the best, the rest will follow. Eat well, not too much, avoid sugar and fat. The Mediterranean diet is a good option, fish, poultry, vegetables, fruits, whole grains, beans, nuts and olive oil. Red meat preferably once a month. Drink natural water, avoid bottled soft drinks. Take care of your appearance, always clean, clothes in good condition, well groomed, polished shoes. Try to eat at your grandparents' or parents' house as long as possible. Do not drink alcohol, if you decide to do so, do it after the age of 21, and never get drunk. Do not smoke, and never use drugs such as marijuana, cocaine and others. Practice exercise, walk 30 minutes a day is enough, run, swim, do weights, soccer, basketball, volleyball, are good options. Read, in books is the wisdom of life, cell phones, tablets only to communicate, study or work. Listen to music, if it is classical the better. Try to play an instrument, the guitar is a good choice, just for that you will be welcome wherever you go. When you start working, give the best of yourself, with enthusiasm and discipline from the first day. Never offend and much less hit a woman, always protect her. If you meet a woman respect her, and if you want her to be your partner in life, take care of her, love her, pamper her. If you have children, remember that you will be their example. Never make fun of anyone. Be kind to everyone, rich or poor, wise or ignorant, sick or healthy. It is in bad taste to swear, avoid it. Respect older people, they have the experience and good judgment that can help you. Do not be shy, be honest, authentic, congruent, between what you do and what you say. One way to understand these issues is to think of our task in life as becoming who we are. You are somebody, you can take your life. Do well to become who you are, rather than denying yourself, or distorting yourself, and never getting to know yourself. In reality, you don't know who you are right now, but you have an idea. And over time, that suspicion may grow until they become more and more sure of themselves. It's not guilt to want to live a quiet life. Let money not be the goal of your life. More important is that they live in peace. You do not need to be heroes. Look at what gives you meaning, what you believe will give your life its deepest meaning. Put your efforts there. You will come to the conclusion that conventional success is not real success, not even for conventional reasons. Success is having served and done good. Find comfort within yourself, not outside. Remember to always be grateful to God, to your parents, to life, show that you are well born.

NOTES ON MEDICINE IN THE CITY OF SAN FRANCISCO DE CAMPECHE

It is of great interest to review some notes on the history of medicine in San Francisco de Campeche. The first hospital was the Hospital de Nuestra Señora de los Remedios, which became the Hospital de San Juan de Dios, later it was the Hospital Manuel Campos, whose name still persists. Dr. Manuel Campos was a pioneer in medicine, he was formed next to the Spanish doctor Dr. Antonio Frutos, he was in charge of attending with care and wisdom the cholera epidemic that affected Campeche in the previous century. In the present time a reference is Dr. Nazario Victor Montejo y Godoy who was a milestone in medicine in Campeche, besides being a cultured person, scientist, poet, attending patients from San Francisco de Campeche and Camino Real, being recognized as a good doctor of great humanism. He taught classes at the Benemérito Instituto Campechano, anatomy, botany, zoology, famous was his museum where he had, flora and fauna of our state. He was a prolific writer and among his writings were his books "Humoradas y Mi Odisea", which fortunately were published by the Universidad Autónoma de Campeche. In the middle of the last century, a group of doctors from Campeche wishing to continue their specialization studies decided to go to Cuba, such as Abraham Azar Farah, the brothers Luis and Jorge Gonzalez Francis, Alvaro Vidal Vera, who among them cooperated to support their families, who stayed in Campeche, They stayed in Campeche to train in various specialties such as ophthalmology and otorhinolaryngology, orthopedics and traumatology, urology, since moving to Mexico City was an adventure, due to the distance and the lack of good communication, it was difficult to travel by boat to Veracruz and from there by train to Mexico City. Other doctors did manage to move to Mexico City, among them Dr. Longinos Apolinar Amabilis who specialized in Surgery, being Dr. Gustavo Baz Prada his tutor. Dr. Erbe Hurtado Estrella, also in Surgery. Dr. Javier Buenfil Osorio who specialized in Pediatrics, performing the first venoclysis, which was a turning point in medicine in Campeche, saving lives, since dehydrations were treated with "papers" which were medicines wrapped in paper, ingested orally, with great morbidity and mortality.It is worth mentioning Dr. Francisco Berron Navarrete, the first psychiatrist in Campeche, who specialized in the Hospital de la Castañeda, also in a tutelary capacity. Dr. Ignacio Guerrero Ramos, gynecologist and obstetrician with his clinic at Maternidad Santa Teresita. Doctors who, without having academic training, but tutelary as Dr. Victor Rivero Alvarez, who practiced urology, Dr. Fernando Herrera Escalante, radiologist. Dr. Hernán Quijano Herrada, dermatologist, who thanks to him the School of Medicine became a Faculty, dermatology being the first specialty with university recognition.

After them, doctors arrived in Campeche who had their first formal training in hospitals. An example of this is Dr. Rodolfo Romero Gutiérrez, who specialized in gynecology and obstetrics in Cuba, and other doctors from Campeche who returned to the state. Among them we have Dr. Pablo Montero Flores with specialty in Orthopedics and Traumatology who performs surgery in favor of the most vulnerable population with the support of Dr. Luis Iglesias de la Torre, of the same specialty, Cuban.At that time, let us remember Dr. Eduardo Rivas Cervera who had his sanatorium in what is now the Obispado, Dr. Salvador Pacheco López, gynecologist and obstetrician. Of good memories. Dr. Ramón Rodríguez Barrera, pediatrician, who started the campaign against the human immunodeficiency virus infection, which contributed to destroy myths and fears about this disease. Dr. Luis Vera Esquivel, otorhinolaryngologist, who was Municipal President of Campeche.

Dr. Fernando Sandoval Campos, Dr. Rufino Sosa Almeyda, Dr. Tiburcio Puerto Parrao, Dr. Joaquín Aguilar Rodríguez, Family Doctors. And, other salubrious physicians in what was called Coordinated Public Health Services, such as Dr. Carlos Miguel Vargas, Dr. Wilberth Escalante Escalante. Some of them are no longer with us and others, fortunately, are still with us. To mention just a few, such as Dr. Pedro Lara y Lara, Dr. Antonio González Coba, Dr. Carlos Talango Poot, Dr. Miguel Medina Maldonado, Dr. Ermilo Novelo Zapata, Dr. Omar Arceo Cárdenas who have gone before us along the way. Others continue as Dr. Octavio Arcila Rodríguez, Dr. Gabriel Díaz Licon, Dr. Miguel Ángel Vargas Rubio, Dr. Manuel Gantús Castro, Dr. Gaspar Ortega Zurita, Dr. Wilberth Brito Burgos, Dr. Alberto Ruiz Rodríguez, Dr. Carlos Acuña Rosado, Dr. Carlos Acuña Rosado, Dr. Carlos Acuña Rosado, Dr. Carlos Acuña Rosado, Dr. Carlos Acuña Rosado and Dr. Carlos Acuña Rosado. Dr. Carlos Acuña Rosado. Dr. Manuel Gracián Barrera, who founded the current school of medicine. How not to remember doctors who gave luster in the different municipalities such as Dr. Eduardo Baeza Garcia, Dr. Pedro Suarez Cardenas of Calkini, Dr. Ernesto Azcuaga del Valle, Dr. Mario Pacheco Hidalgo in Hecelchakan, Dr. Janell Romero Aguilar in Hecelchakan, Dr. Janell Romero Aguilar in Hecelchakan and Dr. Mario Pacheco Hidalgo in Hecelchakan. Dr. Janell Romero Aguilar, Rufino López López of Escárcega. In Carmen Dr. Socorro Quiroga Aguilar, Dr. Rubén Ortega Quijano, Dr. José del Carmen Ferrer Hernández, Dr. Raúl Gutiérrez Arias. In Champotón Dr. José Nazar Raiden Dr. Jaime Amaro Morales. In Tenabo Dr. Olvera Hita. In. Palizada Dr. Jose Lastra Garcia, Dr. Nelson Glory Escofie. In Hopelchén Dr. José Guerrero Barahona, Dr. Fernando Méndez Mejenes. These are just a few, surely there are more, who have given all their knowledge and humanism for their patients. It is important to mention the first woman physician, Dr. Omersinda Ortiz Treviño who worked as an epidemiologist. Dr. Melba Amaro de Vargas, wife of Dr. Carlos Miguel Vargas, and we cannot forget Dr. Yolanda Quijano Argaez, who for many years attended only women in her office.

It is worth mentioning that in Campeche, in the middle of the last century there were no health institutions, so the Unión Médica was formed by doctors Luis González Francis, Javier Buenfil Osorio, Salvador Pacheco López, Fernando Herrera Escalante, Fernando Sandoval Campos, Manuel González Quijano, Roque Buenfil Blengio, Manuel Ramos Quero, Ramón Rodríguez Barrera, Jorge González Francis, among others, which gave rise to what today is the IMSS. Time went on and health institutions arrived, such as the Secretaria de Salubridad y Asistencia in 1944, the Instituto Mexicano del Seguro Social in 1957, and the Instituto de Seguridad y Servicios Sociales de los Trabajadores del Estado in 1975. Currently in Campeche we have excellent doctors from Campeche and other parts of the Republic who have enriched medical science, all of them good medical professionals, humanists. And, a School of Medicine, pride of all of us, that has given us magnificent doctors who have put on a high level the name of Campeche, both nationally and internationally, and institutions that care for the health of all of us.

DESIGNER BABIES

Recently there has been a news item in the media, a controversy about the scientific case of He Jianki, from the South China University of Science and Technology, who claimed to successfully edit the germ line of two girls to avoid the transmission of the genes responsible for the transmission of the human immunodeficiency virus. In 1932 the book Brave New World was published by Aldous Huxley, in this novel the development of reproductive technology was proposed, at that time science fiction, in the XXI century it seems to become a reality with gene therapy. To prevent diseases such as Fanconi's anemia, a rare hereditary disease, umbilical cord stem cells have been used. In recent years, scientists have discovered a new technique that for the first time makes it possible to quickly and precisely alter, erase and rearrange the DNA of almost any organism, including our own, putting a new and dangerous capability in the hands of mankind. The case of a human embryo living in a laboratory dish, where scientists verified that it did not have Fanconi's anemia, in order to treat the sister who had Fanconi's anemia. This has caused controversy, since there are those who say that a baby can be designed according to its needs, eye color, skin color, height, weight, etc. This has been rejected by religious, governmental and non-governmental organizations. And, although gene therapy is already a reality, it must be administered under bioethical criteria. Not everything that is technically possible is ethically and legally acceptable. The creation of designer babies is not limited by technology, but by biology: the origins of common traits and diseases are too complex and intertwined to modify DNA without avoiding introducing unwanted effects. As is the case that the gene encoding red hair increases the risk of skin cancer. In He Jiankui's analysis of gene-edited babies, by trying to make the babies resistant to HIV, they could have an increased susceptibility to West Nile virus or influenza infections. The inevitable rise of designer babies was heralded in 1978 after the birth of Louise Brown, the first invitro fertilization baby, as the next step toward a world where parents can select The same situation occurred in 1994, when a 59-year-old British woman pushed the limits of nature by giving birth to twins using donated eggs that were implanted in her womb at a fertility clinic in Italy. Thus, like many other biotechnological and scientific discoveries throughout history, this genetic engineering procedure raises transcendent ethical questions such as: playing God, genetic discrimination, distributive justice, commercialization, eugenics. What is truly fundamental is that all the social, environmental and ethical implications can be discussed on the basis of serious and rigorous information, which must be provided by scientific experts, jurists, bioethicists, etc. Free of prejudice. Information, education and transparency are the pillars on which the decisions that a society must make about its future must be based.

BENEFICENCIA

Medicine, science of uncertainty and art of probability.

William Osler (1849-1919)

It is here where the health professional has a leading role, for example the physician who makes decisions based on evidence and inferences, sometimes by dogmas, such as this is so because it has always been so, because my teacher says so, because it is published in such and such journal; or by deductive inference this must be so, because the current physiopathological or pharmacological knowledge foresees it; or inductive inference this is so because I have seen it in many other similar cases; besides what is currently in vogue the scientific evidence based on evidences. The physician makes the diagnosis based on the clinic, his knowledge, his personal experience and the data reported to him by the laboratory. He informs himself, thinks, decides and acts. For this it is essential that he has reliable information; he makes the decision based on the information provided by the laboratory. Remember Weinstein and Fineberg, nature is probabilistic, information is incomplete, outcomes are valuable, resources are limited and decisions are inevitable.This is why the principle of Bioethics, beneficence, which consists of considering the need to evaluate the advantages and disadvantages, risks and benefits of the proposed treatments or research procedures, with the aim of maximizing the benefits and reducing the risks, must be borne in mind. It has a positive dimension, which implies the unwavering duty to carry out specific actions aimed at procuring the well-being of individuals and defending their rights, preventing harm and eliminating conditions that generate risk, discomfort and pain, among others. This principle of beneficence is of great relevance.The health professional should offer the best, be updated, attend teaching activities, participate in medical and biomedical research, in order to give the best of himself. The physician, or the patient, requires the services of the laboratory, sometimes it is unknown how professional a laboratory is, if it is updated, if its staff has a code of ethics, if they have principles and values such as honesty, integrity, justice, confidentiality, efficiency, cooperation, legality, dignity, trust, leadership. The physician requests several analyses, trusting fully in the work of that laboratory, it is difficult for him to know a priori how it works. The patient does not know whether the health care professional, doctor, nurse, chemist, social worker or otherhealth professional is up to date in knowledge and skills, not doing so commits fraud with the patient.

If we were asked to define "well-being", most of us would say something like "feeling happy" or "feeling good". We tend to associate our well-being with positive feelings, such as excitement, hope, pride or gratitude. But, for many of us, these feelings are fleeting and have no lasting effect; positive feelings are only one element and, in fact, they are the weakest element. Five elements of well-being have been described; **Positive Emotion, Engagement, Relationships, Achievement, Meaning.** Positive emotion; we all want to experience positive emotions because it simply makes us feel good, enjoy a good meal, go to a party, buy a new dress or have a cocktail on a beautiful beach. Positive experiences trigger all sorts of chemical reactions in our bodies and we feel good. Positive emotions feel great but they don't last long. However, many psychologists see positive emotion as a weak element of overall well-being because it is short-lived. Many studies have shown that the side effects of positive emotion are minimal. A delicious meal or a good movie will make you feel brilliant at the time, but it won't make you feel happier the next day. The other elements of well-being have been shown to have much longer lasting effects, such as **engaging** in activities that require our full concentration, everyone is different, so everyone's activity will be different, writing, playing an instrument, playing a sport, an interesting hobby or project at work. **Relationships** are incredibly important to our well-being, study after study has shown that people with strong relationships have better physical and emotional health. The number of relationships is not important, it is the closeness of the relationships that matters. People with many casual friendships are likely to suffer from loneliness much more than people with only one very close relationship. Having at least one person with whom we can share our innermost feelings helps relieve stress and avoid depression. Good friendships make us happier. **Achievement** Nature was smart enough to realize that if we were not rewarded for our accomplishments, we would get nothing done for the day and risk being eaten by lions. Therefore, every time we accomplish something, our brain releases dopamine, which gives us a surge of satisfaction, to enhance our well-being: We can't rely only on seeking positive feelings. We need to strive for engaging activities, emotional relationships, finding a deeper purpose and pursuing meaningful goals, giving **meaning** to our life.

BIOETHICS

What is bioethics? It is a branch of applied ethics that reflects, deliberates and makes normative and public policy approaches to regulate and resolve conflicts in social life, especially in the life sciences, as well as in medical practice and research, that affect life on the planet, both now and in future generations. Bioethics, without being a code of precepts, integrates analytical activity and is based on philosophical principles and scientific criteria, in order to guide practice in the different areas of health and research, promoting the safeguarding of human dignity and human rights. Medical ethics, why? The study of ethics prepares health professionals to recognize ethical dilemmas, difficult situations and to deal with them in a rational and principled manner. Ethics is also important in the physician's relationship with society and colleagues and for the conduct of medical research. What is the role of bioethics in medicine? Bioethics constitutes an essential support for the resolution of dilemmas that may arise in any health care process, as well as in the interaction between health personnel, patient, family and society in general. The practice of medicine can sometimes go beyond the strictly clinical sphere, which is why it is necessary to form interdisciplinary groups that can evaluate cases and the prospects for solutions from different points of view and provide advice. How should physicians behave ethically with patients? It is important that physicians know and demonstrate by example the core values of medicine, especially compassion, competence and autonomy. These values, along with respect for fundamental human rights, serve as the basis for medical ethics. Compassion, competence and autonomy are not unique to medicine. However, physicians are expected to exemplify them more than others, including many other types of professionals. The physician-patient relationship has been radically reframed. Previously the physician acted and the patient complied, but today the patient's right to decide on the course of treatment is recognized. As well as the physician's ethical and legal obligation to provide the patient with all relevant information about his or her disease and treatment options. The physician must preserve health, cure, or when it cannot be alleviated, always comfort, accompany the patient and avoid premature and unnecessary deaths.

PARTICIPATORY BIOETHICS

Transforming health systems and promoting initiatives that contribute to overcoming exclusion, inequity and barriers to access and timely use of comprehensive health services is a task for all those involved in the health sector. Forty years after the Alma Ata declaration, no progress has been made in combating inequity in health care, and various mechanisms have been accentuated, such as the segmentation and fragmentation of health systems. This has resulted in people receiving medical care depending on their place of work or their ability to pay out-of-pocket, which means that those with more resources have access to better services. In addition, there is a multiplicity of medical infrastructure, which has led to the centralization of the treatment of ailments, instead of attending to the individual's health in a comprehensive manner. In daily medical care there is a doctor-patient relationship, most of the time satisfactory, although sometimes it is not so, breaking that relationship either by negligence, imperfection or imprudence. And many times due to a lack of humanism and communication. The physician is a depositary of trust, an advisor, someone to whom to turn to in any circumstance, in any event, and not only in those related to physical ailments. The physician participates to accompany, to advise, to help. Medicine is the most human of the arts, the most artistic of the sciences and the most scientific of the humanities (Pellegrino). Every medical act has risks, from an aspirin (bleeding) to a complex surgery such as transplants (host versus graft). The duty of the physician is to minimize the risks, as far as possible to control them and above all to establish direct communication with the patient, so that he/she understands and consents to what is going to be performed on him/her. The medical act must be practiced by the medical professional, subject to the rules of professional excellence in force (Lex Artis Ad Hoc), taking into account the scientific development, the complexity of the medical act, the availability of equipment and means of work, and the specific circumstances of the patient's disease. Considering the bioethical principles of the medical act such as: Autonomy which is the respect for the decisions of the informed patient, who has the right to decide about himself, according to his life plans; Beneficence which privileges the good of the patient; Non Maleficence (primum non nocere), Hippocratic aphorism where the obligation of not causing harm was pointed out more than 2000 years ago; Justice, desired by all, where all are treated equally, regardless of race, age, religion, social position. Currently, it has been observed that when there is a bioethical dilemma in a medical unit, in order for it to be addressed, it must be in writing, so that it can proceed. Some members of hospital bioethics committees (CHB),bioethical cases that arise, but since the intervention of the CHB is not requested, they do not get involved, arguing that, although guidance is given, sometimes the patient or the service provider does not wish to express it. This is probably due to our ancestral culture of accepting any situation, without demanding their rights, this is observed mainly in public hospitals, where the care given is considered a favor, fearing that, if they make known any ethical situation, they will no longer be attended as they should. That is why the member of the CHB must get involved with the patient, let him know that he is not alone, that he will accompany him in his bioethical dilemma. At present, bioethics is centered on hospital bioethics committees (CHB) and research ethics committees (CEI), patients and health-related personnel, their function being rather contemplative, although their main functions have been described as being consultative, guiding and educational. The aforementioned at their express request. It is here where the members of the CHB and CEI, should participate in an active way when they become aware of a bioethical dilemma that affects dignity. Privileging autonomy, the protection of human rights and justice. It is in the CHB, where a prudent solution is proposed. It does not sanction, it is not deontological, it establishes recommendations, based on the study of the ethical dilemmas that arise in clinical practice and teaching in the hospital environment. Hence the importance of its members being participatory. Hospital bioethics committees are preventive. Bioethics should not be focused only on standards of good clinical and research practices; it is more than a contemplative bioethical approach. We must build a bioethics for all. To achieve this, the State Bioethics Commission will have a policy of intervention, making bioethics a reality, making pragmatic the right to health protection as a social guarantee enshrined in the Political Constitution of the United Mexican States. By identifying and systematizing the elements that affect a bioethical issue, in order to offer relevant information about them to institutions, social groups or any other sector interested in the subject at the state level. (Creation Agreement 19 05 2008). Therefore, members of public and private hospital committees will be asked to intervene when there are bioethical dilemmas. Once the seed of bioethics is sown, it will begin to bear fruit, it is everyone's task.

BIOETHICS AND HUMAN RIGHTS

Everyone has the right to a standard of living adequate for her or his health, well-being, food, clothing, housing, medical care and social services, as well as the right to social security, maternity and child care and assistance, and the right of children to social protection. To this end, the Universal Declaration on Bioethics and Human Rights was signed in Paris on October 19, 2005. This international instrument shows the need to consider the right to health linked to bioethics. Bioethics and human rights are guarantors of the survival of humanity. But rights are more than dry and legalistic phrases. To the extent that it represents giving legal meaning to the values we hold most dear, dignity, respect, equality. When we see justice done, an intense emotion arises from the depths of all good men and women. That is why society requires for its development, instances of communication, dialogue, agreement and negotiation between different groups and social actors, as well as between these and the State, to analyze and discuss the ethical, legal and social problems that emerge as a result of making Human Rights prevail. Bioethics arises from the need for a bridge between science and humanism. These movements contribute to transforming the healthcare space, user satisfaction in medical services as a criterion of quality of care. The bioethical culture is aimed at awakening in individuals and society the need for a conscious and growing moral development, in order to face in a rational and well-founded way the uncertain situations of social development and the application of scientific and technological advances. The Universal Declaration of Human Rights came to define the most complete ethical project that humanity has, which is common to human beings, human dignity. Within the framework of human rights, the protection of health has been established as a constitutional right. Human Rights and Bioethics have the same purpose, the regulation of social conduct in order to protect basic ethical goods, such as knowledge, freedom, personal integrity, equality, justice, equity, cultural diversity, solidarity, cooperation and health.

BIOETHICS AND TRANSPLANTATION

An act of love

Bioethics is considered the branch of applied ethics, which reflects, deliberates and makes normative and public policy approaches to regulate and resolve conflicts in social life, especially in the life sciences, as well as in medical practice and research that affect life on the planet, both now and in future generations. Sometimes transplants are bioethical dilemmas. Currently, due to the lack of transplants, many people die while waiting for an organ to restore their health. Since long ago, there have been awareness campaigns about transplants, slogans such as "kidneys are not buried can save lives" and other similar ones. However, in 2016 in Mexico there were 20420 patients waiting for an organ, of these kidney 12477, liver 377, heart 49, cornea 7486. Of these only 33.3 % had been transplanted, hence the ethical importance that entails the importance that the population is aware of organ transplantation, since they can restore health. Let's do good, let's try to transplant. Organ transplantation, one of the medical miracles of the 20th century, has extended and improved the lives of hundreds of thousands of patients worldwide. Scientific and clinical breakthroughs by dedicated health professionals, as well as numerous acts of generosity by organ donors and their families, have made transplantation not only a life-saving therapy but also a shining symbol of human solidarity. However, although the action of transplantation is noble, it is limited, either for cultural or religious reasons, causing illegal practices such as transplant tourism in countries like Thailand. For this reason, the Istanbul Declaration was made in 2007, which establishes to guarantee the protection and safety of living donors and the adequate recognition of their heroic performance while fighting against transplant tourism, organ trafficking and commercialization of transplants. Given the importance of transplants in 2010, in Aguascalientes, it was established that the fundamental bioethical principles that should be contemplated are dignity and beneficence, integrity and non-maleficence, precaution and/or vulnerability, autonomy and responsibility, distributive and local justice. Therefore, the vulnerable population must be protected, in this case the poor who for economic benefit offer one of their organs such as the kidney, unethical situations in transplants that promote inequality and exploitation of people, where it is not the poor people in need of money who benefit from the sale of their organs, but rather the intermediaries of this type of sales who get richer. It is clearly defined that it will be the poor who are most at risk of participating in this type of procedure because of their vulnerability.The situation of polarization of the distribution of wealth, the high rate of poverty and the low level of schooling, make it necessary to take the necessary measures to protect the vulnerable population from these new forms of human exploitation such as the trafficking and commercialization of organs. Bioethics has had a particular relevance since the beginning, mainly in the definition of death criteria and in the optimal conditions for the realization of transplants, regarding equity in the access to transplantation, criteria for the allocation of organs from deceased donors, safety of the living donor, risk of commercialization practices, access to immunosuppressive drugs. At present, organ transplantation systems must continue to be perfected, improving the training of professionals and the population, with greater quality and excellence. This is everyone's task.

CHOCOLATE

Do you like chocolate? The following is interesting, there is evidence that dark chocolate can lower blood pressure, total cholesterol and LDL cholesterol and increase HDL cholesterol, which may represent an effective strategy in the prevention of cardiovascular disease. Dark chocolate is derived from cocoa beans, which are rich in polyphenols, specifically flavonoids that have antihypertensive, anti-inflammatory, antithrombotic and metabolic effects, which contribute to cardioprotection. The ingestion of dark chocolate promotes relaxation of the arteries, lowers blood pressure, improves endothelial function, decreases interleukin 3, interleukin 1B, and the level of Von Willebrand factor. An important fact is that after 4 weeks of chocolate consumption, a decrease in circulating leukocytes was observed, which suggests a lower inflammation, since leukocytes can migrate through the endothelium and play a primary role in atherosclerosis. Dark chocolate intake is associated with better cognitive performance and improved structural integrity of brain white matter in patients with cardiovascular risk factors. Furthermore, dark chocolate contains theobromine, an alkaloid found in the cocoa tree, which increases urine production, due to its diuretic effect and vasodilatory ability. The word 'theobromine' originates from (Teo-dios, joke-food), or the food of the gods, chocolate is the final product of the processing of the fruit of a tree popularly called cacao. The Mayas used cacao as currency. In Campeche it was and still is traditionally taken mixed with water for breakfast. Its ingestion produces wellness, let's avoid the white chocolate that is presented in different commercial presentations and that the advertising media recommend it for being tastier, because of the amount of sugar and fats it contains, which can cause harm. Do not forget that chocolates should be consumed in moderation, dark chocolate gives 376 calories per 100 grams. Caution, let's take care of our intake and calculate the calories we need according to our activity.

UNIVERSAL HEALTH COVERAGE, FOR EVERYONE, EVERYWHERE

The most precious thing a human being has is health. Our Political Constitution establishes that every person has the right to health protection. The World Health Organization establishes that health is a state of complete physical, mental and social well-being, not merely the absence of disease or infirmity. It is a fundamental human right, and the attainment of the highest possible level of health is an extremely important social objective worldwide, the realization of which requires the intervention of many other social and economic sectors in addition to health. Governments have an obligation to care for the health of their people. In 1978 in Alma Ata, Kazakhstan, in the most important health policy event in the world, "Health for all in the year 2000" was established, 40 years have passed and it is still a longing. In several countries, including our own, there is a fragmented health system, different health institutions, public and private health care. In an attempt to unify health services, towards a universal health system, the policy of "universal health coverage for everyone everywhere" was established, where quality medical care and humanism must be received. For this reason, since 2001, public policies have been developed in our country to bridge the gap in health care, to provide health coverage and protect the population against catastrophic expenses derived from it, and thus promote the constitutional mandate of the right to health protection for all Mexicans, which in the paragraph added to article 4 stipulates: "Everyone has the right to health protection". The right to health is not the same as the right to health protection. It is appropriate to point out that the former is broader, while the latter seems to account, rather, for the obligation of the State to develop positive actions aimed precisely at protecting health or repairing it when it has been affected. On April 7, 2018, the World Health Organization, calls on world leaders to commit to concrete actions to promote the health of all people through universal health coverage to be achieved when there is strong political determination. This means ensuring that everyone, everywhere, can have access to essential, quality health services without financial hardship. No one should have to choose between good health and other necessities of life. For health services to be truly universal, it is necessary to move from health systems built around diseases and institutions to health systems built around and for people. So that "Health for all" becomes a reality and not just a wish.

COMFORT, COMFORT

A word of encouragement, to comfort an afflicted person, is to comfort, a word that in these days acquires a special meaning, when a son cannot say goodbye to his father, to give him a last hug, because of the pandemic that we have had to live and that has left uneasiness, fear, uncertainty. And, many t i m e s , the only thing left to do is to console, to comfort. There is nothing more human than to support those in need. The human being needs to be comforted, how many times in his desperation sometimes tries to take his own life, when the only thing he probably needs is to be comforted. In this era of modernity where values have been lost such as effort, honesty, honor, respect, integrity, well doing. Now what matters is what has value, the acquisition of material goods, social position, no matter how they are obtained, e i t h e r by corruption, dishonesty, how to comfort those who are afraid of losing their health, economic resources, without despairing even more those who have none? These questions are even more acute today as the current pandemic increases fear. That is why empathy must be present. To rejoice life and comfort the spirit is to inject new energies to achieve tranquility in this new normality. To comfort, to comfort those who have lost a loved one, from whom sometimes they have not said goodbye, giving rise to a shock that is limited to a certain degree of kinship, parents, grandparents, siblings, friends. Mourning for the loved one has gone from being an intimate and familiar mechanism of symbolic mediation. It has become part of a statistic. Living with the pandemic is always possible, even most people do it, they comply with health measures. However, living well, which for many means contributing to the environment a greater added value, for example, when going on vacation, they forget about preventive measures, causing their health and those around them to deteriorate. Sometimes desperation sets in. So comforting has a human meaning, by committing to help the sick person in the search for the meaning of his suffering, because when he has an idea about that meaning, when that human being puts himself in the shoes of that suffering human being, he will understand it. Accompanying the sick person in this search for meaning in his suffering is the commitment that we should all have with our fellow human beings. The sick person, who seeks health, who asks above all for a warm help, a comfort, for his ills, his ailments, which, even if they are physical, affect his spirit. He still feels neglected, tragically and painfully ignored and abandoned. It is when he needs to be comforted. To comfort is not simply a pat on the shoulder; sometimes this is more like pity than anything else. It is to understand, to help the one in need. In order to achieve an authentic humanization, in those moments in which theMperson feels fragile and distressed because of illness. Cure sometimes, relieve often, comfort always.

INEQUALITY

Nothing hurts more than inequality, and this is present in all social, educational, health and economic spheres. We should all have the same opportunity to have access to achievements, but in reality this is not the case. If we review the social rights contained in legal documents, in the International Covenant on Economic, Social and Cultural Rights, we observe that there must be a remuneration that provides as a minimum to all workers: fair and equal pay for work of equal value, without distinction of any kind; in particular, women must be assured conditions of work not inferior to those of men, with equal pay for equal work, decent conditions of existence for themselves and their families, Safety and health at work; equal opportunity for all to be promoted, within their work, to the superior category that corresponds to them, with no other considerations than the factors of time of service and capacity, rest, enjoyment of free time, reasonable limitation of working hours and periodic paid vacations, as well as remuneration for holidays. This covenant must be complied with. As well as the existence of good or desirable states of affairs such as the right to a clean environment or to enjoy the benefits of scientific progress or cultural heritage. Many countries are in agreement with the above and they are in their laws and decrees, but the dilemma is who guarantees it? In theory, they should be applied in a unitary manner based on the interdependence and indivisibility of all civil, political and social rights, both in axiological and structural terms. Emphasizing the guarantee of rights. Human rights, an obligation with regard to those responsible for protecting them, both institutional and extra-institutional. Social rights are human rights, i.e. rights that we all possess by the very fact of belonging to the human race. Let us say no to inequality, and let us strive for equality, which means that all human beings are of equal value and should be treated equally, regardless of their ethnic origin, sexual orientation or ability. Human rights must be more than wishful thinking, they must be applied primarily to those who have the least, the voiceless, the vulnerable. Education is the guarantor that inequality does not exist. Without the active participation in favor of equality of all, both women and men, whether in the educational, health, economic or political areas, it will not be possible to reduce social inequality.

TEACHER'S DAY

Teacher's Day is a holiday that honors the work of teachers. May 15 is a very special day, a day of celebration, to recognize all those who throughout time have offered their talent, ingenuity and effort for the sake of teaching. There is nothing nobler than the vocation of teaching. The teacher who in a give and take amalgamates with the student. Giving the best of himself, to form better women and men. How much dimension exists when the destiny is teaching, and this is perhaps the most complex and transcendent destiny, because to devote oneself to the difficult task of teaching requires passion, but above all, vocation. He who sacrifices himself for the good of others, who guides his students towards the conquest of knowledge through teaching that moves, the truth that moves, the energy that galvanizes, has to be a teacher of a great destiny, and thus with the strength of this passion for the truth and freedom of man, moving great obstacles, to build day by day a lasting work, the work of the transformation of man, in the professional that society requires. Teaching is a task that requires a profound structure of knowledge and full conception of teaching; of knowledge, because it is the basis and foundation, of teaching, because it is motivation and dynamism. And, in this mixture, we understand that the student requires intellectual and physical freedom; to realize himself as a human being, it is evident then, the need to understand him, and thus, with the intensive force of judgment, to guess the pearl of intelligence that seemed to be hidden in the student's conscience here is where the teacher and his deep intuition, makes him give his life, where his individuality becomes plurality, where he lives for himself and for others and thus enter the colossal world of true teaching. This is precisely the difference between the mediocre teacher and the successful one, between the ordinary and the extraordinary, because positive results are the consequence of work, dedication, effort and motivation. It is important to know, but more important than knowing, is knowing what to do with what you know. Knowledge is a treasure that provides happiness to the extent that it is transmitted and that without the pleasure of communicating it, knowledge would mean nothing. The teacher's reason are the students, restless and indifferent, respectful and disrespectful, responsible and irresponsible, assistants and absentees, restless and serious. Those who transmit us their problems and their achievements, their encounters and misunderstandings, the complicated and the happy, those who protest about everything and those who question everything, and when they want to, they rival and challenge us. All this is part of the profile of these exceptional and beloved beings, called students. Students who today are the nodal part of the intellectual task. The teacher's permanent commitment is to continue questioning ignorance, to reproach indolence, to reject the superfluous, to turn each student into a new man and to achieve in him, transformation, evolution, change in the rhythm of his own history.

INTERNATIONAL DAY OF WOMEN AND GIRLS IN SCIENCE

The International Day of Women and Girls in Science, celebrated on February 11, was proclaimed in 2015 by the United Nations. According to UNESCO between 2014 and 2016, only about 30 percent of all female students chose higher studies within the field of science, technology, engineering and mathematics. For centuries women have been discriminated against by not allowing them access to education, work, the arts. Yet there have been women who have made significant contributions in the fields of science and art. They have discovered life-saving drugs, humanized care for the sick, inventions that have improved the world, far-reaching research, contributed works of art in music and painting. But in many cases their invaluable advances are minimized. Women's work has changed the way we see the world. That is why, on the International Day of Women and Girls in Science, let us remember some women who have made the world a better place. Sor Juana Inés de la Cruz, Mexico's first feminist, who had to enter a convent to write her poems and books. Matilde Montoya, the first physician, who after many obstacles managed to enter the National School of Medicine, in those years of the nineteenth century, which suggested her to dedicate herself only to housework. Florence Nightingale, forerunner of the professionalization of nursing today, her actions in the Crimean War inspired the formation of the Red Cross, she is still remembered in the Ceremony of the passing of the light in the faculties and schools of nursing when they finish their professional studies. Marie Curie, physicist and chemist, winner of two Nobel Prizes, discovered two elements polonium and radium, which are the basis of X-rays, and radiotherapy in the treatment of cancer. Tu Youyou, Chinese pharmaceutical chemist, who discovered artemisinin for the treatment of Malaria, being awarded the Nobel Prize in Medicine in 2015. And, Dr. Celia Alpuche Aranda, from Campeche, who obtained in 2019, the national research award, for her contribution in bacterial pathogenesis, epidemiological and molecular mechanisms of antimicrobial resistance. Let us remember the words of Mae Jemison physical engineer and NASA astronaut. "May you never be limited by the limited imagination of others".

DIGNITY

"Human beings are WORTHY, because they are human beings, not because they have the same values or share the same beliefs."

Diego Gracia

Are you a worthy person?

Most people will say yes, but will we be worthy of it?

Just because we are human? How many times this dignity is not respected by ourselves, when we accept perks, let alone if there is corruption. Quite a lot has been said about dignity; from the definition of dignity by the Royal Spanish Academy of the language, followed by institutional statements, all speak of dignity. From the lat. dignĭtas, -ātis.1. f. Quality of dignified.M2. f. Excellence, enhancement. Gravity and decorum of persons in the manner of behaving. Dignity, or The term "quality of dignity" (from the Latin: dignĭtas, which translates as "excellence, greatness") refers to the inherent value of human beings simply because they are rational beings, endowed with freedom. Article 1 of the Universal Declaration of Human Rights, adopted by the United Nations on December 10, 1948, begins with the following statement: "All human beings are born free and equal in dignity and rights". From this perspective, the dignity conferred by the status of being a citizen is nourished by the republican valuation of an orientation towards the common good. This brings to mind the meaning that the ancient Romans gave to the word dignitas; namely, the prestige of statesmen and public servants in the service of society. Although, of course, the distinction accorded to a few exceptional "dignitaries" and a few notables contrasts with the dignity that the constitutional state must guarantee to all citizens equally. According to Kant everything has either a price or a dignity. That which has a price can be substituted by something else as equivalent; on the other hand, that which is above all price and therefore admits of no equivalent possesses dignity. All human beings are born equal in dignity and rights and, endowed as they are with reason and conscience, must behave fraternally towards one another. The universal declaration of human rights came to define the most complete ethical project that humanity has, which is common to human beings; the essence of these rights is human dignity. To be treated with dignity and respect by patients and their families, as well as by the personnel related to their work, regardless of their hierarchical level. All these statements speak of dignity, but the reality may be different. Sometimes dignity is not valued. This is something that should not be accepted, especially by physicians, since the patient comes to them in search of help, comfort and dignity, which is often lost in hospitals, it seems, for example, when a woman is a victim of obstetric violence. If there is a human right that should prevail is that of dignity, that is why saying that dignity is useless, is to say that the essence of the human being is useless. Therefore, dignity is to attend the patient with delicacy, courtesy and conscience. Dignity is to provide adequate and pertinent information so that the patient can make a decision. To propose alternative solutions and seek them in their case. Charge fees for service according to their ability to pay, the importance of the service provided and the means used for it, provide an environment of trust, comfort and hope, and if possible next to their loved ones. To treat him with patience, constancy, tolerance and prudence. To be loyal to him and zealous guardian regardless of his circumstances, regardless of his origin, skin color, sex, religious belief, civil status, sexual preference, economic situation, social position, state of cleanliness, odor or pathology. It is dignified to console him when science exhausts its resources and to accompany him in his last breath...It is dignified to show respect for his right to dignified treatment. Physicians must protect the dignity of patients and be indignant when a patient's dignity is not valued. We must raise our hands and speak up for those who have no voice. We can and must do something, and this is solidarity with all our brothers and sisters regardless of social status or skin color. Is dignity related to poverty? It would seem so. If the patient is poor, indigenous, he is referred to as you, he is looked down upon, he is discriminated against. Does dignity have to do with justice, it would seem so. If the patient is vulnerable because of his color, economic status, he is treated in a way that is not fair, not dignified. Let indignation serve to build the foundation of our ethics of conviction, commitment and responsibility. The worst thing that can happen to a human being is to be stripped of his dignity. To be dignified is to be a person, a person of integrity, integrity, honesty, who when he or she reaches the end can say that he or she was a dignified man or woman.

END-OF-LIFE DILEMMA, ADVANCE DIRECTIVES, ADVANCE DIRECTIVE

Death is inevitable, a bad death is not.

A dilemma arises, there is the possibility of extending life or prolonging the arrival of death, it must be decided to what extent and how to intervene, since all power must have certain limits, and therefore this situation must be approached in such a way that respect and protection of human rights and dignity is maintained at all times. It should not be overlooked that the conception of death is intimately related to other cultural constructs, and that in this sense the way we think about death depends on the way we understand the value of life and what it means to protect and sustain that value. Given the current relevance of the discussion of the main dilemmas at the end of life due to technological advances and the rise of a new paradigm around the care of terminal illnesses, the development of palliative care and the attention that has been paid in the legal sphere to respect for autonomy and other human rights, it is essential to deepen the current state of the debate on this issue. Currently, there are several states in the country that have an Advance Directive Law at the end of life, such as Mexico City, Coahuila, Aguascalientes, San Luis Potosi, Michoacan, Hidalgo, Guanajuato, Nayarit, Guerrero, State of Mexico, Oaxaca, Yucatan and Tlaxcala. These States are concerned about human dignity in the last stage of life and in some cases take into account the social problem of unnecessary expenses. In general, they prohibit behaviors that result in the intentional shortening of life; they do not intend to promote euthanasia, but rather to recognize the right to refuse therapeutic treatment and to receive so-called palliative care. It is important to mention that most of the state laws mention elements related to ethical dilemmas at the end of life, and indirectly promote organ donation and transplantation. The Law of Advance Directives at the end of life is not mandatory; it is an option for those who wish to do so. The purpose is that people can live according to their condition as human beings at the moment of their own death, without someone else making decisions for them. We are not talking about a dignified death, but about a dignified life until the last moment. This means not only the elimination of pain and suffering, but also respect for autonomy, that is to say, the will about the type of care one wishes to receive and up to what moment. It is anchored in the collective unconscious to face death, this is an individual experience, which depends on the vision that each person has of himself and of life. Above all, the dignity of the person is safeguarded at all times until the last moment of his or her life.Unrestricted respect for personal decisions in accordance with their beliefs, values, principles, dignity and human rights is fundamental.

MEDICAL DILEMMA

An elderly man with coronary artery disease, who lives with his wife, who is also 80 years old, has frequent unstable angina at night. When this happens, he is taken to the hospital, where he stays for a few hours and is discharged. His physician assesses the situation and finds that from a cardiological point of view, the expected benefit of further hospital admissions is minimal, while the burden of anxiety and the disruption caused by the transfers is terrible for both elderly. After a prudent and understandable discussion with the patient, his wife and close relatives, the patient decided that the angina would be treated at home. Probably the decision taken has favored a course of action that will surely result in a better quality of life for the elderly man. Technically and legally it would have been correct, and of course more comfortable for the physician, to continue recommending admission for successive episodes of unstable angina. However, the overall quality of the decision taken in this case, which includes ethical criteria (weighing the elderly person's preferences), was possibly superior. This is where the physician becomes involved with the patient. Some will say don't get involved with the patient, is that an ethical dilemma? No, because the patient comes to the doctor in search of help, of an anchor, a bridge to help him, of someone who understands him, of a human being. Let us remember that medicine is service. That is why we must take the patient by the hand and guide him/her through the sometimes rough and winding path that is the disease, and it is not enough to make an accurate diagnosis and an effective therapy, it is something more and it is our duty as physicians to accompany this affected organism and desolate soul. The statement that one of the forces that should move physicians to improve the quality of their practice must be ethics is certainly true. But it is also true that this statement often remains just wishful thinking. We must be humanists in order to participate in the change we all desire, if by humanism we mean love for our fellow man. Let us be responsible for that human being that looks for us, for his relief, remembering that we help with what we know, not with ignorance. Let us be active, proactive, committed. Let us not forget that health in its broadest concept, as defined by the World Health Organization, is the complete state of physical, mental and social well-being and not only the absence of disease. Therefore, it is necessary that health reaches every corner of the country, where there are committed physicians, creative officials who reduce the deep inequalities. That is why when we treat a patient, let us not be satisfied with just making a good diagnosis, a timely treatment, let us do something more, as in a give and take, where the patient and the doctor amalgamate, let us shake hands with the patient and together we walk the path with a deep human sense full of love and understanding for our patient. A human being who requires inMoccasions just a few words of encouragement. So there is much more to do.

ETHICAL DILEMMAS SURROUNDING MIGRATION

There is no path on foot, the path is made by walking

Antonio Machado

One of the most difficult situations that humanity presents is migration, reasons why people have always migrated, to escape war, persecution, discrimination, to find better opportunities and get out of poverty, to seek better opportunities, to support their families and build a better life. Migration has been present since the dawn of humanity, this phenomenon is increasing. Therefore, preserving the health of those who migrate or emigrate; protecting their dignity and rights and safeguarding their lives both now and in the future, is a crucial and priority task. The migrant's right to health is closely related to the exercise of other rights, such as the right to protection against all forms of violence, to food, to housing, to decent work, to education, to non-discrimination, to access to information. In this task, bioethics is a fundamental tool for decision-making in this regard. By pointing out the ethical challenges such as: Who provides health services? Who finances these services?

How can compensation mechanisms be established, how can the resident population be protected alongside the migrant population? It is here where bioethics must permeate the analysis and the search for solutions to such complex phenomena as migration, from a solidary, secular and inclusive perspective. What is the best way to manage resources in the face of scarcity?

What is the best way to address inequities, what is the best way to solve the social determinants of health, the determinants of preventable losses in the quality of life or well-being of populations? Sometimes the migrant is alone, he/she is vituperated, denigrated, our population sometimes experiences this when migrating to other countries and even more so if he/she is undocumented. The same happens with migrants from other countries when they arrive in our country. Mexico is an example of migration, and how it has helped the migrant, if we remember the last century with the Spanish migration, product of the civil war in that country, and Campeche itself, welcoming migrants fleeing from neighboring Guatemala, due to insecurity. Campeche has been an example of support to migrants by establishing medical units for their attention. Campeche is a state of transit, destination and origin of migration, it is a migratory corridor where there is an important challenge in providing access to health care to the migrant population. If we do not understand the phenomenon of migration, it is a return to barbarism, it is condemning us to even the most primitive of human beings. Therefore, society has the ethical responsibility to provide health care and protect the health of undocumented migrants, people who were not invited to the country but who showed up there and work there. At In the case of migrants, marginalization is unacceptable, and reducing inequities in the case of health is an ethical imperative.

ABSURDITY IN MEDICINE

Why?

In the practice of medicine absurdities are observed, first let us define what we mean by absurd, according to the dictionary of the Royal Spanish Academy, contrary and opposed to reason, that makes no sense, extravagant, irregular, shocking, contradictory, irrational, arbitrary or nonsensical saying or fact. The absurd is a concept that refers to irrational thought, the opposite of rational thought, which departs from reason and behavior. Extravagant, the opposite of behavior considered normal or conventional Albert Camus (1913-1960), writer, philosopher, makes known the philosophical ideology of the absurd, in his book L'Étranger this book is the product of socio-political conditions of a time, as was the 2nd World War, when Germany invades France, the question arises why? It is an absurdity, contrary to reason, that men kill each other. As physicians, we often observe absurdities, when we are students and we have the idealism of humanism, we ask ourselves the question "Why? Doctors who become merchants, untrained doctors, unethical doctors, and at the end of the day, many become this absurdity. It is absurd the lack of access to quality health services in poor populations, the abuse of transnational companies that promote obesity, mainly in unprotected populations, being absurd that poor people are overweight, since the thrifty genes, make this overweight is mainly fat, and not protein. To die young is an absurdity, as well as at the end of life with suffering and without dignity. In medicine it is absurd that there are maternal deaths, children with malnutrition, women victims of violence by those who should protect them, cancer patients who cannot obtain medicines, medical schools that do not respond to a social demand but to a desire for profit, doctors who make their profession a business, where the desire for economic gain predominates. Humanism and ethics are in the way. Suicide is an absurdity, it goes against the reason to live, and the absurdity of the obligation to live when it is no longer desired, but society prevents it. How many times we witness the absurd and we do nothing, it is easy to be in the comfort zone. It is our duty to do what is necessary to avoid absurdity, unreason. An ethical question that we should all apply. The philosophy of the Absurd seems to be somber. Already Camus argues that we must all recognize the absurd, searching for its meaning. In this sense, for Camus, what is absurd is the confrontation between the call of man and the unreasonable silence of the world.Physicians should act according to their principles and values, in order to avoid absurdity. Although there are a great number of absurdities, the following principles should be followed. The teachings obtained mainly in the family, the teachings of good teachers. Recognize that the absurd is not an expression of defeat, nor is it an excuse not to give the best of oneself, as a doctor you must continuously train in knowledge and skills. Absurdity must be confronted, and although it is exhausting, a passionate effort must be made to be better. Absurdity exists and is present, it is our duty to prevent it from persisting, that is why we are physicians, with the question "Why?

THE MEDICAL ACT

In daily life, few acts are as transcendent as the medical act, and it is the relationship between two beings, one who needs help and the other who provides it. Being a physician is an attitude of service to the human being, procuring physical and mental well-being, preventing disease, promoting health, relieving pain, caring for the sick who have no cure, preventing premature and unnecessary death, helping people to die well. One is a doctor to help another human being, the doctor is the depositary of a trust, which should not be defrauded, the doctor must offer the best of himself, in knowledge, in skills. He is par excellence a humanist. The physician is a human being, and as such can make mistakes. Medicine is not an exact science, as Dr. Pellegrino said, medicine is the most human of the arts, the most artistic of the sciences and the most scientific of the humanities. Every medical act has risks, from an aspirin (bleeding) to a complex surgery such as transplants (host versus graft), the duty of the physician is to minimize the risks, as far as possible to control them and above , all to establish direct communication with the patient, so that he/she understands and consents to what is going to be performed on him/her. The medical act must be practiced by the medical professional, subject to the rules of professional excellence in force (lex artis ad hoc), taking into account the scientific development, complexity of the medical act, availability of equipment and means of work, the specific circumstances of the patient's disease. Considering the bioethical principles of the medical act such as Autonomy which is the respect for the decisions of the informed patient; he has the right to decide about himself, according to his life plans, Beneficence which privileges the good of the patient, Non-maleficence (primum non nocere), Hippocratic aphorism where he points out more than 2000 years ago, the obligation to do no harm, Justice desired by all where everyone is treated equally, regardless of race, age, religion, social position. We should all be co-responsible for health, a decision should not be made solely by the physician instead of the patient nor by the patient independently of the physician. Rather, the decision should involve the physician and the patient. The physician should make decisions for and with the patient, not meaning the "for" instead of the patient but in the patient's interest. And, on the other hand, the virtue of integrity, which refers to the values we cherish and defend, such as honesty and respect for human rights. Co-responsibility in health care is shared between the patient and the patient.

PAIN RELIEF, A HUMAN RIGHT

"Only he who suffers it, knows what he feels."

Pain has accompanied mankind since the beginning of time. According to the International Association for the Study of Pain, pain is defined as an unpleasant sensory or emotional experience associated with actual or potential tissue damage, or described in terms of such damage. There are different types of pain. Three main types of pain have been described: nociceptive, neuropathic and psychogenic. Nociceptive pain is the body's normal response to an injury and is intended to prevent further damage (e.g., removing the hand from a hot object after the first contact). On the other hand, neuropathic pain such as diabetic neuropathy, and psychogenic pain which is real and requires psychiatric treatment. Pain is therefore subjective and exists whenever a patient says that something hurts. The World Health Organization (WHO) declares that: "chronic pain is a disease and its treatment is a human right". And, in its statement of the concept of health. WHO defined health as "a state of complete physical, mental and social well-being and not merely the absence of disease or infirmity." Pain is a serious public health problem worldwide, its management is sometimes not adequate, either for various reasons from religious ones that accept pain as a divine punishment, or from professionals not prepared to treat pain. Living without pain should be a human right, and not only human, but of every living being. In our country, the General Health Law suggests the opening of spaces for the attention of patients in the field of pain and palliative care. It is necessary to train the health team in pain management, liberalization of national policies on the availability of opiates, supported by a health system that allows equitable access to medical care and appropriate drugs. And, thus fulfilling the goals of medicine, which are to preserve health, to cure, to relieve, to comfort, to prevent premature and unnecessary deaths. Pain is a problem all over the world, the effective management of acute and chronic pain is not always adequate and sometimes not available to everyone. Therefore, pain relief should be considered a human right, although the transition from the current concept of pain relief as an aspiration and a right to be defended, to a future in which pain relief is a universal reality, will require a great deal of effort, commitment and vigilance.

GOOD AND EVIL

How can we explain that a human being attacks another human being, steals his belongings or his life? The drama of Auschwitz in Nazi Germany is a before and after in all fields, especially in the field of thought, the magnitude of evil has been such that humanity has become mute in the face of such horror. Once again, human action has put the fragility of good to the test. Can man seek evil? Yes, everyone desires the common good, good health, good finances, good personal relationships. However, there is evil, when there are lies, theft, rape, crimes. Is the human being evil by nature? A newborn with its genetic load is neither good nor bad, neither goodness nor badness is inherited. It is known that he is born with characteristics that are inherited by the father and the mother. It is the environmental conditions that influence between goodness and evil. When there is an action of evil it denies the human condition, human dignity, since it always considers the other, through the systematic use of violence, as a means, as an object and never as an end in itself; therefore, it destroys human nature as a possibility. To think of the possibility of evil comes from conceiving man as capable of good and evil, as indeterminate, which can lead him to the highest degree of perfection, to a happy and solidary existence, or to his destruction. The good has to do with everything that is thought, willed and done because it is considered good. The good, therefore, possesses objectivity beyond what is recognized. It is not a being, but a value that we recognize not by knowledge, but by intuition. We intuit, we know what is good, there is a sentimental perception that pushes us to prefer, to love the good. Evil can always be overcome by good If evil can be the end of an action, this would be an active faculty governed by destruction, that is to say, essentially negative. Can man seek to destroy himself and the society of which he is a part? On many occasions it does, and mankind has witnessed this. That is why, from early childhood, children must be cared for. It is not possible for child abuse and street children to exist. International organizations such as the United Nations (UN), have established since 1989, the Rights of the Child: Children are persons and subjects of law, they can and should express their opinions on issues that affect them. Their opinions must be heard and taken into account for the political, economic or educational agenda of a country. In this way, a new type of relationship is created between children and adolescents and those who make decisions on behalf of the State and Civil Society. The life and quality of life of children must be preserved, guaranteeing their harmonious physical, spiritual, psychological, moral and social development, taking into account their aptitudes and talents. No child should be disadvantaged in any way for reasons of race, creed, color, gender, language, caste, situation at birth or for having any kind of handicap. physical. Humanity has the capacity to do good. A very thin line separates good from evil, everyone is responsible for what they do in the end.

STRESS IN THE TIME OF THE PANDEMIC

In these days of SARS-CoV2 pandemic, where stress is present every day in health personnel, fearing infection and consequently the family, or the family of the sick person who when admitted to the hospital does not know if they will see their loved ones again. Stress wreaks havoc on the organism. In 1936 Hans Selye [1] demonstrated that stress generates hypersecretion and hypertrophy of the adrenal glands, as well as atrophy of the thymus and lymph nodes. It is considered as "General Adaptation Syndrome. Stress cannot be avoided, since it is a biochemical reaction, but it can be controlled. Stress is a normal component of our life. The stress response has been evolutionarily selected to cope with environmental threats that endanger our survival. For our ancestors, stress was a clear advantage, since it was necessary to obtain food, reproduce, defend themselves, find shelter. Stress can increase adrenaline and cortisol, these hormones when activated, mobilize stored energy to the muscles, which causes an elevation in heart rate, blood pressure and respiratory rate, while disabling metabolic processes such as digestion, reproduction, growth and immunity. Cortisol reduces ATP (adenosine triphosphate) production and increases inflammation. When you have a stressful situation, it cannot be avoided, for example, if you win the lottery jackpot, or your car is stolen, you will have a stressful situation with the release of hormones such as adrenaline and cortisol. Hence the importance of having a healthy organism. A good diet is essential. If you do not nourish your body properly, you will not have the vitamins and minerals needed to produce enough ATP, and you will feel more tired. Eating too many processed foods can increase inflammation, which impairs ATP and energy production. If you are eating too much food at once, that can cause blood sugar spikes and lead to fatigue, so eat whole foods, such as vegetables, fruits, whole grains and lean proteins such as fish, chicken, nuts and seeds. Prefer smaller meals with snacks in between to provide your body with a steady supply of nutrients and fewer blood sugar spikes. The Mediterranean diet [2] has been recommended, which is characterized by a high intake of vegetables, fresh fruits, legumes and cereals, olive oil. Moderate alcohol consumption, mainly in the form of red wine during meals no more than one glass, fish, moderate dairy intake and eating red meat once a month. People may have high cholesterol and this can lead to atheroma plaques in blood vessels, such as the aorta, carotid arteries, hence the importance of controlling lipids. Since the situation may arise when there is stress and the release of hormones, mainly adrenaline and cortisol, which can destabilize the plaque and release a part of the atheroma that can migrate to different organs such as the brain and cause a thrombotic event with the [3] For what is fundamental the feeding and the exercise. It has been recommended in the courses of self-control of stress, that when you feel stressed squeeze as hard as possible the fingers and toes, so that the action of hormones is in the lower limbs and not in vital organs. This accompanied by relaxation techniques such as yoga, Tai Chi.Avoid inactivity. If you are sedentary, you may have less muscle mass, which leads to fewer mitochondria and less ATP. Being sedentary compounds the problem by weakening and shrinking muscles and causing them to use energy inefficiently. Physical activity strengthens muscles, helps them become more efficient and conserve ATP, and increases the production of energy-producing brain neurotransmitters. Don't be intimidated by the recommendation of 30 minutes per day, at least five days per week, of moderate-intensity exercise. The 30 minutes can be spread out over several shorter periods. It can be simple, such as climbing stairs or walking farther in a parking lot.Lack of sleep [4] increases cortisol and also promotes inflammation. If sleep problems are caused by sleep apnea (pauses in breathing during sleep), decreased blood oxygen levels decrease ATP and energy. Talk to your doctor about underlying problems that may deprive you of sleep, such as health conditions (sleep apnea or frequent trips to the bathroom) or medication side effects. And try to improve your sleep hygiene, go to bed and wake up at the same time every day, and keep your bedroom cool, quiet and free of electronics, which stimulates your brain.Avoid sugary soft drinks as they can cause blood sugar spikes followed by a drop that causes fatigue. In addition, excess sugar can lead to obesity and disease such as diabetes mellitus. Being dehydrated can also make you feel tired, as can drinking too much alcohol or caffeinated beverages close to bedtime (alcohol interrupts sleep in the middle of the night). Stress can also affect the immune system by decreasing its function, which can prolong the time it takes to treat the disease [5].If stress cannot be avoided, it can be controlled, for this we must have a healthy organism, especially in times of pandemic, where stress control is fundamental.

References

1. De Luca, Sanchez M, Perez O, Leijas S. Comprehensive measurement of chronic stress. Mexican Journal of Biomedical Engineering;25: 10.
2.	Trichopoulou A, Lagiou P. Healthy traditional Mediterranean diet: An expression of culture, history and lifestyle. Nutr Rev 1997; 55/11:383-389.
3. Fuster V, Thrombus remodeling: key point in the progression of coronary atherosclerosis. Revista Española de Cardiología 1999;53(51):2.7
4. Vela Bueno A. Olavarrieta Bernardino S, Fernández Mendoza J. Sleep and stress: relationship with obesity and metabolic syndrome Rev Esp Obes 2007; 5 (2): 77-90.
5. González Gómez B. Escobar A. Stress and Immune System. Rev Mex Neurosci 2006;(1):31-38

THE PHYSICIAN PUBLIC SERVANT AND ETHICS

Where business begins, the decorum of the profession ends

Dr. Ignacio Chavez

The physician is considered a public servant since he/she is a person who provides a service of social utility, in addition to caring for the health of the population, he/she must act ethically, considering this as the set of moral standards that govern the conduct of the person in any area of life. The most important duty of physicians is to provide care that is in the best interest of patients. With up-to-date knowledge and skills, failure to do so is unethical. Physicians serve society, in this case the public. Their ethical performance has been observed since time immemorial, few professions are as closely watched as that of physicians, since the time of Hippocrates. To this end, codes and norms have been written about the principles and values that physicians should have as public servants, including honesty, legality, loyalty, impartiality, efficiency, and values such as public interest, respect for human rights, equality, non-discrimination, equity, gender, cultural and ecological environment, integrity, cooperation, leadership, transparency, accountability [2]. The physician as a public servant must also have compassion, understood as understanding and concern for the suffering of his fellow man and empathy, which refers to the cognitive ability to perceive, in a common context, what another individual may feel. It is also described as a feeling of affective participation of one person in the reality that affects another. Empathy means knowing how to appreciate feelings, in other words "put yourself in their shoes". For these and many other things, we owe it to the people. At the end of the medical career, the Geneva Declaration of the World Medical Association is made

> ➢ I solemnly promise to consecrate my life to the service of humanity,
> ➢ To give my teachers the respect and gratitude they deserve,
> ➢ To practice my profession conscientiously and with dignity,
> ➢ To look after my patient's health first and foremost,
> ➢ Keep and respect the secrets entrusted to me, even after the patient's death,
> ➢ To uphold, by all means in my power, the honor and noble traditions of the medical profession,
> ➢ To consider my colleagues as brothers and sisters,
> ➢ I will not allow considerations of age, illness or disability, creed, ethnicity, gender, nationality, political affiliation, race, orientation, gender identity, gender identity, gender identity, gender identity, or gender identity to be taken into account in my decisions. sexual, social class, or any other factors come between my duties and my patient,
> ➢ To ensure the utmost respect for human life,
> ➢ Not to use my medical knowledge to violate human rights and civil liberties, even under threat,

➢ I make these promises solemnly and freely, upon my word of honor.

If most of us physicians are convinced of the above, what is happening, why are patients mistreated, why is there arrogance, negligence, commerce, why do these situations arise? Why is it that over the years, instead of caring for the human being, the golden calf is worshipped, it is mercantilism that prevails. As the distinguished Master Dr. Ignacio Chávez Sánchez used to say, where business begins, the decorum of the profession ends. The physician shall live well with his income, but not with insulting fortunes based on the pain of a fellow human being. Being a physician demands not to prostitute the profession with the indecent trade of his services. In the Greek Olympus, where all promiscuity was permitted among the gods, who even used to come down to earth in search of the love of mortals. Hygeia, later elevated to goddess of Medicine, never shared the thalamus with Hermes, god of those who live by trade. Any improvement in the performance of physicians and public hospitals towards greater efficiency will only be possible if the morale of public servants is raised through proper ethical training. It is important that physicians working in public hospitals have a comprehensive training with values and principles, with a sense of responsibility, loyalty to the patient and to the institution. Commitment to themselves to offer the best of themselves.

THE POWER OF MEDICINE

In January 2016, a renowned physician sexually assaulted a black female patient, (1) at one of the most prestigious academic hospitals in the US. IT HAPPENED RIGHT IN THE EMERGENCY ROOM, A PLACE HE WENT TO IN HOPES OF RECEIVING CARE. It happened right in the emergency room, a place she went to in hopes of receiving care, and initially no one believed her. When semen analysis showed that she was, in fact, right, that this doctor had drugged her and proceeded to ejaculate on her, many questioned how this could have been possible.To most, this would seem even more surprising and not credible. Perhaps his power, prestige and sense of invincibility were all factors that really made him feel he could get away with exploiting others. How many similar cases are known, physicians who are considered the non plus ultra, these exist in most hospitals. There have been reported cases (2) of abuse, sexual and otherwise, most of the time nothing happens.e know that power in medicine has created and perpetuated obsolete hierarchies, which has led to abuse not only of patients, but also of medical students and other health professionals. What about academia in medicine in training programs, medical residencies, too many physicians with too much power and too little oversight to keep that power in check. While any physician could harm a patient or colleague, those who are exceptional in their fields are probably more immune to the consequences. If physicians have the potential to become abusive, why do they do it and how might we stop it? Some have pointed to the growing epidemic of burnout and among physicians-in-training as contributors. In one study (3), researchers found that medical students who were more "burned out" were more likely to behave unprofessionally and with less humanism in caring for patients, especially vulnerable ones.Another reason may be that we are not selecting the right type of people to be doctors. In Mexico, medical admissions systems are geared to test scores, which means that a doctor with good grades is excellent for medical school. But that doesn't necessarily translate into what patients often consider important: a doctor who listens to them, cares, has empathy and treats them as an equal partner. Research has shown that emotional intelligence can be helpful (EQ). In contrast to IQ. Some medical schools are changing to change their admission criteria to better reflect this need, but most do not.But aside from these reasons, we should not underestimate the fact that power inherently corrupts, especially when there is no system in place to keep it in check. Many of the prestigious physicians who have gotten away with harming others have been protected by their institutions.At Yale Medical School (4), a physician remained director of his research institute and was invited to return as head of his division after sexually harassing students. The reality is that reputable physicians are important to reputable institutions. Some bring in large amounts of research grants; others increase the influence and prestige of the place where they work. But the people in charge who have the power to do something about abuse should ask: Isn't a patient's safety worth more than saving prestige or protecting research money?

Patients deserve the best doctors, but the best doctors are not always the most famous doctors. When it comes to helping, the patient will not care how many titles are behind the name of their doctors, how many publications, awards. When illness strikes, they will want someone to be by your side, holding your hand, treating you with respect and care and recognizing that they are a human being. Doctors who think they are God will not be able to do this. We don't need more powerful doctors in medicine, what we need are good doctors.

Bibliography

1. One night at Mount Sinai, Aja Newman went to the emergency room for shoulder pain. Her doctor was a superstar. What is the worst that could happen? The Cut Oct 15 2019
2. Harassment and discrimination in medical training: a systematic review and meta-analysis. Fnais N , Soobiah C , Chen MH , Lillie E Acade Med F , 2014 May; 89 (5): 817-27. doi: 10..1097.
3. Changes in Empathy during Medical Education: An Example from Turkey
4. Artiran Igde Pak J med Sci 017 Sep-Oct; 33(5): 1177-1181
5. Yale Medical School Removes Doctor After Sexual Harassment Finding
6. The New York Times, 14 November 2014

PREGNANCY AND ADOLESCENCE, AN INJUSTICE

There is nothing more unjust than stealing the innocence, the hope of a girl, an adolescent, and this injustice is present in our country, in Campeche. According to the Manual of Adolescence of the Pan American Health Organization (PAHO), adolescent pregnancy is the gestation that occurs during the two years after the onset of menarche when the adolescent maintains total social and economic dependence on the parental family. The marriage of girls is a particularly dramatic reality. Worldwide, it is estimated that every three seconds a girl is forced to marry; 14% of girls living in developing countries, such as ours, will be married before the age of 15. The backwardness of inequality and discrimination experienced by most adult women is the result of a perverse circle; girls are the women of the future, they are educated for a society where women are discriminated against; educated to live for others; educated to be women in a society where women are the "other" discriminated against, without rights or with limited rights. The greatest risk of maternal mortality corresponds to adolescents under 15 years of age, where complications of pregnancy and childbirth are the main cause of death in most developing countries. To prevent maternal death, it is also essential to avoid unwanted pregnancies or pregnancies at too early an age. According to the latest data published by INEGI in Campeche the percentage of registered births to teenage mothers under 20 years of age is 19.4, counted up to 2015. The entity ranks number seven, the first place nationally is occupied by Coahuila and the last one by Mexico City. The negative sanction hinders access to information, education and preparation to exercise sexuality in a pleasant and responsible way, so that much of the problem lies in the way adults qualify the phenomenon; in the way social institutions, family, school, religious institutions, the health sector, etc., interpret and handle it. We must take care of girls, they are our future. Avoid early courtships that occur from the age of 10, which many parents accept and see these early relationships with good eyes, probably in many cases they lived a similar situation. Women should live their childhood, adolescence and adulthood to the fullest, not doing so is often a drama. Education, and in this case sex education, is indispensable. That girl that we all love, parents, brothers, grandparents, must be correctly oriented in the years of adolescence, probably a particularly special situation, since it is the awakening of the senses, the libido. Hence the importance of sex education. To make them aware that at that stage their priority is to study in order to form a patrimony. They should finish their education, start working and with what they earn they should help their family, if that is the case, and buy items of their choice, clothes, perfumes, cars, etc. Once they have children, what they earn will be for them first, then for the house and finally for her. It is essential to take into account the cultural context and the special characteristics of the family to better understand the situation of the adolescent, to support and care for her, especially the parents, and to avoid saying yes to everything, just to avoid problems at home. Children are a responsibility.

WE WERE DOCTORS

We were doctors, people who prepared ourselves to give the best of ourselves, to relieve the sick, not only physically but sometimes emotionally. Nowadays, there is a lot of writing and lectures about the dehumanization of medicine. The commerce of medicine. Doctors who charge $ 1500.00 pesos (66 dollars) per consultation while the minimum wage is $172.87 (8 dollars) 2022) 1 is medicine for the rich? Where poverty represents 43.9 of the population according to INEGI (2022) 2 A country where, thanks to public education in universities, the tuition fee to study medicine ranges from $1000 to4,000 pesos a year. Forgetting that thanks to the population via taxes they managed to become doctors. Adding to this the mistreatment of patients, something is wrong. When the doctor, from a good cradle, should honor, be grateful to those who through their efforts managed to study, and have a profession from which they will live. The poor who do not have economic resources should not be charged, and those who have sufficient resources should be charged according to their work, all this in an ethical manner. One is a doctor not to become a millionaire, one is a doctor to help, and not to get rich through human pain. It is therefore important to remember the words of Dr. Ignacio Chávez (Ideario 1997) 3 Colegio Nacionali "Where business begins, the decorum of the profession ends", "Being a physician demands not to prostitute the profession with the indecent commerce of its services. In the Greek Olympus, where all promiscuity was permitted among the gods, who even used to come down to earth in search of the love of mortals. Hygeia, later elevated to goddess of Medicine, never shared the thalamus with Hermes, god of those who live by trade." "Medicine without science is only a trade, and the physician who remains in it is no more than a simple craftsman".To speak of the commerce of medicine, of dehumanization, from the time of Hippocrates to the present day. Where sometimes the golden calf that is money is worshiped. Forgetting the Doctor who was prepared to help and not to get rich. Therefore it is important to remember the prayer of the Jewish physician Maimonides 4 Make me modest in everything except the desire to know the art of my profession. Let me not be deceived by the thought that I already know enough. On the contrary, grant me the strength, the joy, and the ambition to know more every day. For art is endless, and the mind of man can always grow".Little progress has been made in this aspect; many times they are like the words of John the Baptist, who proclaimed in the desert, words are carried away by the wind. That is why the physician must become human, as was the physician of yesteryear, the family physician, the family doctor. Bioethics, the ethics of medicine must be a pillar in medical education. Nowadays, the more specialized medicine becomes, the more we see a dehumanization, the reification of the patient, commerce. Mainly in the large hospitals known as What happened to the family doctor, the one who was part of the family, who took care of the patient not only physically, but also spiritually. The physician should not forget that if he performs this profession, it is mainly to help a suffering human being. The physician must make decisions for and with the patient, not meaning the "for" instead of the patient but in the patient's interest. And, on the other hand, the virtue of integrity, which refers to the values we cherish and defend, such as honesty and respect for human rights. Co-responsibility in health care is shared between the patient and the patient. Some will say do not get involved with the patient, is that an ethical dilemma? No, because the patient comes to the doctor in search of help, of an anchor, a bridge to help him, of someone who understands him, of a human being. Let us remember that medicine is service. That is why we must take the patient by the hand and guide him/her through the sometimes rough and winding path that is the disease, and it is not enough to make an accurate diagnosis and an effective therapy, it is something more and it is our duty as physicians to accompany this affected organism and desolate soul. The statement that one of the forces that should move physicians to improve the quality of their practice must be ethics is certainly true. But it is also true that this statement often remains just wishful thinking. One must be a humanist in order to participate in the change we all desire, if by humanism we mean love for one's fellow man. Let us be responsible for that human being who looks for us, for his relief, remembering that we help with what we know, not with ignorance. Let us be active, proactive, committed. Let us not forget that health in its broadest concept, as defined by the World Health Organization, is the complete state of physical, mental and social well-being and not only the absence of disease. Therefore, it is necessary that health reaches every corner of the country, where there are committed physicians and creative civil servants to reduce the deep inequalities. That is why when we treat a patient, let us not be satisfied with just making a good diagnosis, a timely treatment, let us do something more, as in a give and take, where the patient and the doctor amalgamate, let us shake hands with the patient and together we travel the road with a deep human sense full of love and understanding for our patient. A human being who sometimes requires only a few words of encouragement. So there is much more to do. That is where we are, for that we need the complicity and support of many other colleagues who, like me, miss being doctors in the genuine sense of the word. It is everyone's responsibility, especially those who train doctors, to ensure that we do not say we were doctors, but that we are doctors.

Bibliography

1. https://www.gob.mx/conasami/articulos/incremento-a-los-salarios-minimos- para-2022?idiom=en
2. Population living in poverty by state according to degree of poverty, 2018 and 2020 (inegi.org.mx)
3. Chávez Ignacio. Ideario 1st Ed. 1997. National College, Ministry of Health. National Autonomous University of Mexico. Ignacio Chávez National Institute of Cardiology.
4. https://www.unav.edu/web/unidad-de-humanidades-y-etica-medica/material-de-bioethics/oracion-de-maimonides

ETHICAL?

Is being ethical old-fashioned? Phrases like "he who does not compromise does not advance", Are they a reality? Before answering, let us remember the illustrious Mexican Jaime Torres Bodet, (1902-1974) "The Mexican of the future will have to correspond to a loyal, honest, clean, energetic and industrious type; Who loves his country dearly, without the need to deceive himself in order to love it, over the evils and weaknesses that still burden it, who is worthy of understanding those weaknesses and those evils, not to exaggerate them with irony or pessimism, but to correct them with work, with sacrifice, with virtue. A type of Mexican that is truthful in everything, truthful with his fellow men, and truthful with himself, faithful to his word, superior to the pettiness of gregarious servility and flattery. A being who does not fold his arms in the face of difficulties, hoping to be saved from them, belatedly, by a stroke of luck, an illegitimate medro, a vile cunning. A being who does not abdicate his rights out of timidity or negligence, but who does not exercise them in an abusive manner either and who, above all, never forgets that the internal guarantee of those rights lies in the fulfillment of duties, because without the fulfillment of duties, any right would result in an exclusive and exceptional privilege. A being who loves life and exalts it. In short, a type of citizen who is capable of judging himself before others, and who knows that above the freedom that is obtained as a legacy, the destiny of the people always places the superior freedom, which is the one that is deserved" Fatherland, I give you the key to your happiness:

Be always the same, faithful to your daily mirror; fifty times is the same the Bird drilled in the thread of the rosary, and it is happier than you...Ramón López Velarde (1888-1921), in Suave Patria. The answer, we are Mexicans, we should be proud to be so. Let us not allow the lack of values to be our common denominator, let us be ethical in the broadest sense of bioethics. Let us be congruent, with ourselves and with society. To be honest, responsible, integral, are values that we cannot renounce. In our country we talk about corruption; is this a habit? No, Mexico is a noble nation in which honest men and women existed and still exist. A nation in which undoubtedly there are many people of integrity. There are more those who think correctly than those who have deviated from the path. Mexico is our country, the country of our parents, of our children, of our grandchildren, for us there is simply no other. Let us love it, let us respect it, this is the only way to make Mexico, so dear to us, what it has always been, a Homeland that welcomes us as a true mother, a priceless treasure of which we are fully proud.

ARTERIAL HYPERTENSION, A SILENT KILLER

In primary health care, blood pressure control is of utmost importance. Its uncontrolled control can lead to hypertension, which affects 18.4% of the population, according to the National Health Survey 2018 in the population over 20 years of age in the country. Achieving good control of arterial hypertension is essential to reduce disability and death from events such as heart attacks or strokes. In Mexico, cardiovascular diseases constitute the first cause of death with 141,619 (INEGI 2018), of which about 30% occur in people who have not yet reached 70 years of age. Arterial Hypertension is characterized by the persistent elevation of blood pressure figures $\geq$ 140/90 ml/Hg. It is important to point out that 47% of people are unaware that they have hypertension. At the beginning there are no symptoms, which is why it is so dangerous. Mexico officially joined HEARTS in the Americas, a PAHO/WHO initiative aimed at improving the prevention and control of arterial hypertension. Campeche was one of the first states where this program was initiated. The program proposes the strengthening of an integrated care model, which reorganizes the tasks and functions among the different members of the health team, including not only medical and nursing staff, but also health promoters, nutritionists and pharmacy staff, among others. It is also important to guide patients in changing their habits to improve physical activity, diet and reduce tobacco and alcohol consumption. It is important to intervene in the causal determinants, starting with diet, since around 30 percent of the cases are related to increased salt consumption and 20 percent to low potassium content in the diet, which translates into low fruit and vegetable intake. We all want to be healthy, let's take care of our blood pressure, for ourselves, our children, our loved ones, let's be co-responsible in taking care of our health.

INCLUDING THE EXCLUDED

"Let no one enjoy the superfluous, as long as someone lacks the strict".

Salvador Díaz Mirón

Sometimes we exclude our fellow human beings, exclusion, as a form of deprivation. The concept of exclusion has proven to be useful, in deprivation and violations of human rights. The language of exclusion is apt and sufficient, as well as the versatility and scope of the concept. Exclusions exist in different areas such as political, economic and social. We exclude those who are not like us. Whether because of economic differences, race, sexual preference or religion. However, there is no conceptual convenience without some cost, and the notion of exclusion is no exception. To see this, it may be helpful to begin by recalling that some of the classic concepts of injustice actually refer to "unfair inclusion" rather than exclusion. For example those who are stripped of freedom of speech or health care are clear examples of exclusion in a way that sweat labor, or being subjected to urban pollution or global warming are present. We should be aware of the two types of injustice, unfair exclusion and unfair inclusion, and should not confuse them. It so happens that many of the most extreme cases of human rights violations, such as the denial of basic freedoms, torture, imprisonment without trial, disenfranchisement and total starvation or lack of medical care, can be well discussed in the format of "exclusion". However, we must also accommodate bonded labor, sweat labor, child labor, environmental affectations, etc., which are seen as unfair inclusion. Indeed, we must also take advantage of the empirical fact that there is often a remarkable congruence of deprivation across various types of exclusions and inclusions for the real underdogs of society. Some citizens are wealthy; most are not. Some are very well educated; others are illiterate. Some lead an easy life of luxury; others are made to work incessantly under terrible conditions. Some are influential; others lack influence altogether. Some have lawyers; others do not. Some are treated with respect by the police; some are not. In fact, most notably, many are often income poor, suffer from illiteracy, work hard in terrible conditions. The dividing line between "have" and "have not" is not just a rhetorical cliché or an eloquent slogan, but, unfortunately, a substantial feature of the world in which we live. The concurrence of different deprivations in the form of congruent exclusions is a general characteristic of the state of human rights. Let there be no unjustly excluded or unjustly included. Let us all have enough to live with dignity, because the dignity is no one's banner, it is everyone's flag, no matter what the economic income, color or religion, and this dignity will be transformed into peace, that peace sought by those who follow Buddha, those who believe in Christ, those who are agnostic. That peace to which all men of good will aspire on earth.

JUSTICE

Justice, from the Latin Iustita, is the conception that each era and civilization has about the meaning of its legal norms, it is a value determined by society, the need to maintain harmony among its members. It is the set of rules and norms that establish an adequate framework for relations between people and institutions, authorizing, prohibiting and allowing specific actions in the interaction of individuals and institutions. Justice is a principle of bioethics, in which it is intended that the distribution of benefits, risks and costs in health care or research be carried out in a fair manner. That is to say that they are distributed equitably among all groups in society, taking into account age, sex, economic status, cultural and ethnic considerations. It also means that all patients in similar situations should be treated similarly and with the same opportunities for access to the best possible diagnostic and therapeutic methods. Justice is a desire to which we all aspire. It is unjust not to provide quality medical care. As well as the waste and squandering of sometimes scarce resources that individuals and society allocate to a valuable purpose such as health. Equity in the distribution of benefits, in patient care and access opportunities, is a requirement of society. If we are to have distributive justice, health-related services have, within a justice delivery model, a greater importance than other goods. How can we satisfy health needs equitably, if the resources to do so are limited? Because people pursue a wide variety of goods, resources to meet health needs will always be limited. To answer this question, it is useful to examine our agreements and disagreements about how to prioritize the distribution of resources to meet health needs. Is justice a common good, a necessity for the survival of humanity, an interesting study carried out at the University of California, in the United States of America, in 2008, where it is shown that reactions to equality are connected in the brain and that equality is activating the same part of the brain that responds to food. This is congruent with the notion that being treated equally satisfies a basic need, Justice.

EMPATHY IN MEDICINE

Empathy from the Greek ἐμπαθής ("moved") is the cognitive ability to perceive, in a common context, what another individual may feel. It is also described as a feeling of a person's affective involvement in the reality it affects.Empathy, from the Greek empatheia, means knowing how to appreciate the feelings of another. The term empathy was introduced in 1909 by the English psychologist Edward Bradner Titchener, as a translation of the German word einfühlung. It was Southard, in 1918, who was the first to incorporate empathy in the doctor-patient relationship, as a facilitating resource for diagnosis and therapy.With respect to the concept of empathy, this is defined as the acts with which the experience of others is apprehended; as Stein expresses, "it is the experience of the consciousness of others in general. It is the experience that a self has of another self, an experience in which it apprehends the soul life of its neighbor".The patient goes to the doctor, not out of sympathy, but because he needs help. It is of no interest to know if the doctor is handsome, with good humor, what he demands is to be restored to health. Let us remember "the family doctor" where the physician is an anchor, a bridge between patient, illness and family. Sometimes, as Antonio Corral Castanedo refers, the patient finds himself on an island, with minimal contact with his family, due to the bureaucracy that prevails in some health systems. When the patient enters the hospital, he is subjected to machines and apparatuses that do not give him any explanation, between analyses and X-rays, explorations that he does not know what they are for and what they are looking for, that stun him and about which nobody clarifies anything, in the midst of which he hears little encouragement, in a few words; he finds himself lost. Doctor Ignacio Chávez already pointed it out in the last century when he warned of technique over clinic, dehumanization, commercial interests, in the search for the golden calf.Empathy, in other words, that the physician puts himself in the patient's shoes. To get involved with the patient not only in the care of the human body, but also in his feelings, his soul, his spirit, everything that makes up the human being as a whole.Why is the physician sometimes no longer empathetic, if the majority of students who wish to study medicine are empathetic, meaning that they wish to help, to be in the patient's place, to understand him/her. What often happens is that this empathy is lost during the course of their studies, whether at the undergraduate or postgraduate level. Therefore, it is important to reinforce empathy in the student and also in the physician who has already graduated. The presence of the mentor must be pointed out, since he is an example for many, and his way of behaving and acting is a paradigm that doctors in training follow. That is why, when starting medical studies, the selection of the future physician must be careful, knowing the principles and ethical values that the physician must have, without neglecting empathy in their training and professional practice.

HOPE AFTER THE PANDEMIC

The word hope has been one of the most used words in these difficult days, with varied purposes and dimensions, such as the scientific hope of the vaccine, the hope of a recovery in health, in the economic aspect. And, the presence of the coronavirus with its fatal effects on health and economy, has led to the greatest desire and longing for hope for a return to normality. Although the road continues at times with a sense of outrage, when the patient is not cared for with COVID, or the vaccines are used in people who are not in the first line of patient care. It is in this devastating, unjust pandemic that we must continue. However, it is good to know that, among so many shadows, there are the lights that appear in this confusing situation we live in. To open our eyes to the need for a humanism of compassion. Mainly to the vulnerable, those who have lost hope, either because of the lack of a loved one, or their economic resources. The ethical principle of protection in the face of vulnerability must always be present. The vaccine has brought new hope and, with it, new challenges. During the darkest months of 2020, while fighting this terrible pandemic, hope in the distance for an effective and safe vaccine brought light at the end of the tunnel. But now begins the daunting task of getting the population protected. Implementing the logistics, as well as overcoming mistrust and fear, now more than ever we must let science guide the public discourse as we try to move forward. If vaccine is wasted, if communities are ignored, if someone can't find their name on a list, something is going wrong. Vaccination has to be done in an effective and efficient way, there is no other way, only this will ensure that vaccines get into the arms of everyone. Not forgetting people with mental health problems, homeless people, people living in poverty, people deprived of liberty, low-income migrant workers, minorities. People with some form of disability, more than one billion people in the world (about 15% of the population). Although progress has been made in their inclusion in society and in equal rights and opportunities, there is still a long way to go to achieve full equity in access to health, education and employment. The public health crisis must not undermine respect for human dignity and the protection of human rights. Therefore, the critical importance of equitable access to vaccination must be emphasized. Considering the challenges facing society, demographic problems, resource scarcity, budgetary constraints, as well as at the same time unprecedented scientific advances, the critical importance of equitable access to vaccination must be emphasized. With regard to vaccination, this means ensuring that everyone, without discrimination, has a fair opportunity to receive a safe and effective vaccine.

MOSQUITO BITES

Why do mosquitoes bite some people more than others? At a meeting, mosquitoes seem to bite only you, relatives and friends as if nothing. It is convenient to know that 20% of people attract mosquitoes in a special way, mainly people of blood group O, and that they are secretors (it is convenient to point out that the person can be a secretor or non-secretor blood group). Mosquitoes bite us to extract proteins from our blood, mainly the female as she needs them to lay her eggs. Another way mosquitoes choose who to bite is by detecting the carbon dioxide emitted in the breath, they use an organ in their jaw and can detect carbon dioxide at a distance of up to 5 meters. Tall people with a larger body surface area attract more mosquitoes than others, which is one reason why children are less frequently bitten. Exercising is conducive to mosquito bites, since substances such as lactic acid, ammonia and uric acid, which are found in sweat and increased body temperature attract mosquitoes. Genes also play a role, as some people sweat more than others, and this can be attractive to mosquitoes. Ingestion of beer and other alcoholic beverages, which make a person attractive to mosquito bites, has been linked to the ethanol excreted in sweat. Pregnant women are more likely to be bitten by mosquitoes because they exhale 21% more carbon dioxide and their body temperature is slightly higher. Another factor is color; mosquitoes are attracted to colors such as black, blue or red. There are people who practically do not get bitten by mosquitoes, this is because they naturally emit mosquito repellents, due to genetic factors that are being studied and are expected to be discovered to avoid mosquito bites.

MEDICINE IS MORE SUBSTANCE THAN FORM

We all remember the family doctor, the family physician, in whom trust was placed. The doctor was like an anchor, to whom the patient and the family clung, until the moment of healing or the fatal outcome. If this happened, the doctor gave comfort to the bereaved and issued the death certificate. The relatives and friends watched over the deceased until it was time to take him/her to the church and then to the cemetery. Nowadays, most people die in hospitals, in a room, surrounded by strangers, with a number on the bedside and their name. Is loneliness the payment to be made in the face of medical progress? Dehumanization? As Dr. Ignacio Chávez commented in his Ideario (1),.... I was so tired! I had done so many surgeries that day! That is not medicine. That is a repair shop, a first class shop if you will, but a shop nonetheless. It is the profession turned into a trade. Sometimes, as Antonio Corral Castanedo (2) refers, the patient finds himself on an island, with minimal contact with his family, due to the bureaucracy that prevails in some health systems. When the patient enters the hospital, he is subjected to machines and apparatuses that do not give him any explanation, between analyses and X-rays, explorations that he does not know what they are for and what they are looking for, that stun him and about which nobody clarifies anything, in the midst of which he hears little encouragement, few words; he is lost. There is the simulation of a doctor who says he is qualified to treat a patient efficiently and effectively, with humanism, but that doctor does not continue studying, does not accompany the patient; and in order to get rich, he offers his services without being up to date in the practice of medicine, forgetting that he studied medicine to help, not to get rich at the expense of the pain of his fellow men. Medicine has had a great scientific progress, there are clinical practice guidelines, official standards, procedure manuals to avoid possible lawsuits. However, there is no law that establishes that the physician must be assertive, empathetic, good-natured, there is nothing worse than meeting a physician who does not smile or does not give confidence. It has been proven that when the patient and the physician, in a give and take, identify with each other, health recovers more efficiently and the physician feels the satisfaction of doing good. Although this law does not exist, which obliges the physician to be affectionate, to sit by the patient's side, to take him by the hand, to say a kind word of encouragement. It should exist. Form and substance in medicine, to be doctors in form and substance. In the form take care of the appearance, the clothes we use, respect the clinical gown, without forgetting hygiene, the doctor must provide confidence. There is nothing more terrible than to find a disheveled, indolent doctor, take care of the way of being a doctor. Basically, this doctor must be up to date in knowledge and skills, so that they can to offer quality medical care. Without forgetting the patient, the family members. Accompanying them at all times from the process of the disease to healing and, if the dying process occurs, showing empathy and compassion. Without forgetting that medicine is more substance than form.

References

1. Chávez Sánchez Ignacio, Ideario. 1st Ed. p. 14. El Colegio Nacional. 1997

2. Corral Castanedo, Antonio. Praise and nostalgia of the family doctor. Commemorative Year of the 250th anniversary of the foundation of the Royal Academy of Medicine and Surgery of Valladolid. 1981.

THE DOCTOR-PATIENT RELATIONSHIP

The relationship between the patient and his physician is based on trust; it is the confrontation of a trust, that of the patient, with a conscience, that of the physician. The doctor has the knowledge and the patient has the hope. In which the patient's well-being will always be privileged. The doctor is the patient's bulwark. Sometimes when the patient arrives at a hospital, he/she finds him/herself on an island, with minimal contact with his/her family, due to the bureaucracy that prevails in some health systems. When the patient enters the Hospital, he is subjected to machines, devices that do not give him any explanation, between analysis and X-rays, explorations that he does not know what they are for and what they are looking for, that stun him and about which no one clarifies anything, in the middle of which he hears little encouragement, few words, he is lost. The doctor, like a lighthouse, points out the light to the sick person, because he longs for someone to look at him, to analyze his state of mind, his shocks, his fears, his loneliness. The sick man, the physical man and as a consequence psychically mutilated, disturbed and diminished, looks for a handle, looks for someone to help him bear and share the anguish engendered by the disease, someone to cure his specific ailment, his own. The doctor as a lifeline will have the kind word that comforts him and his family; the family that spends hours in the waiting room, without knowing anything, anguished over the fate of their loved one. The doctor is the repository of the patient's trust, he expects him to diagnose and treat him, to advise him, but without letting go of his soul and his hand. He must hold tightly that childish hand, that childish existence, in which the life of any patient becomes, no matter how adult and experienced he may be. In the complex, specialized, technified world of today's medicine, amidst the massification of large clinics, amidst the bustle of the big city, of hospitals, passing from waiting to waiting, from queue to queue, from silence to silence, from doctor to doctor. The sick man, the soul of the sick man, who seeks health, who seeks above all a warm help, a consolation, a clarification, for his ills, his ailments, which even if they are physical, affect his spirit, he feels although he is not attended, tragically and painfully ignored and abandoned, he finds in the doctor his salvation. The aim of medicine is the preservation of health and the cure of disease, but also and especially the physical and moral improvement of man and spirit. Every physician must respond to the triple mission of sage in science, priest in purpose and artist in procedure. And, ask God like the Jewish physician Maimonides to desire only knowledge, in order to help his fellow men. That the physician considers his patient in his totality, that he knows his complexity, his personality, in order to successfully reach the recovery of his existential destiny.

SALT

It is ethical for people to know what they are going to ingest.

In Mexico, we love salt, this is a truth, how many of us ingest too much salt, surely a large amount, since we are given to eat a lot of snacks and processed foods, either at parties, going to a baseball game, even at home watching television. The intake of salt can be considered as an addition, since since childhood, we consume large amounts of salt, such as salted peanuts, chamoy, ham sandwiches, processed meats such as salami, just to mention a few. It is recommended by the health system to limit salt intake, however its consumption is high. In statistics from the United States of America, it is estimated that 89% of American adults and more than 90% of children eat more than the recommended 2,300 mg of sodium per day· A similar figure probably exists in Mexico. In Mexico it is common to add salt to food before tasting it. Therefore, it was recommended to food vendors to remove the salt shaker from the table. The major source of sodium is sodium chloride (common salt), of which sodium constitutes 40%. However, all foods naturally contain sodium, the concentration being more predominant in foods of animal than vegetable origin. Diseases such as myocardial infarction, type 2 diabetes mellitus and cerebrovascular disease are related to high sodium intake. The World Health Organization recommends reducing sodium intake to less than 2 g per day for adults. As well as eating fruits, vegetables, seeds. But if you are hypertensive with sodium-sensitive blood pressure, salt can cause negative health effects. Most people consume more sodium than they physiologically need. Salt is necessary, it is true, but it should be limited, one option would be that in foods with high sodium content, there is a legend that says that excessive sodium intake is harmful to health. It is ethical that people should know what they are going to eat, which means that patients should be the ones who ultimately decide on matters that affect them. Their autonomy should be respected.

THE YEARS PASS

Suddenly one turns sixty and, also suddenly, one realizes that one feels the same as at fifty. Suddenly you reach seventy and, also suddenly, you realize that you feel the same as you did at sixty-nine, that is, that turning seventy is less solemn than people think. The elections for the presidency of the United States, to be held in 2020, will feature two candidates who are well over 70 years of a g e : Donald Trump 74 years old, Joe Biden, 76 years old. When you are young, you are young for life, something that I repeat whenever I have the opportunity because it seems to me a truth like a temple, just as it is true that when you are old, you are old from adolescence. Who does not know old and septuagenarian, octogenarian and even nonagenarian young and happy people like Dr. Longinos Apolinar Amabilis, Dr. Guillermo Fajardo Ortiz, Dr. Ruy Pérez Tamayo, just to mention a few. Youth is a fiction that is maintained against all odds, so it is easy to see that true youth, not that of the mere calendar, requires a long apprenticeship. It is only when one gives up being young that old age appears and sweeps away all illusions. I do not deny that being old can be frightening, avoiding euphemisms and jargon, such as senior citizens, full-grown adults, older adults. When in reality they are old, just as there is childhood there is old age. It is all a matter of common sense. The Hungarians say that old age reduces the agility of the horse's legs, but does not prevent it from neighing; the Germans say that the oldest trees bear the sweetest fruit. There is a Harvard University study that concludes that when people are over 70 years old, not only their intelligence improves, but also their happiness increases. Age cannot be a criterion for exclusion and the rules that send the elderly to work paralysis are reactionary. Moreover, discrimination of people on the basis of their age is akin to the segregation of individuals on the basis of their race or sex. At a certain age, all that is needed is to know how to measure distances well and not to ask for the impossible. The bad thing is not getting to be 60, 70, 80 or more years old. The bad thing is not to be able to behave properly and with common sense, that the key to be happy is not to aspire beyond what is reasonable. The first thing that man needs to grow old is to have decorum, that is, to grow old without frivolity and with his feet glued to the ground. At a certain age, all that is needed is to know how to measure distances well and not to ask for the impossible. It can happen to human beings like wine, it can become vinegar or cognac. Whether we end up as a bitter old man who thinks everything is bad, or an old man with empathy, a delight to talk to, depends on us. Henry-Frederic Amiel: "Knowing how to grow old is the masterpiece of the art of living".

THE VOICELESS

Rudolf Virchow's (1821-1902) investigation of a typhoid epidemic in 1848 identified a root cause: "The power of the aristocracy, sustained by the church." Big business is the aristocracy, the politicians, and the church (BMJ 2017; 357:j2996). It has been 169 years now, and the same situation continues, wealth dominated by hegemonic groups, growing poverty, the voiceless. In society's pursuit of wealth and profit, it is the poor who suffer the greatest burden of disease, whose deaths are most likely when fire destroys a village, the levees break. After the Grenfell Tower fire in London, Martin McKee recalls Virchow to urge us not to ignore the political and commercial determinants of public health (doi: 10.1136 / bmj.j2966). Inadequate safety measures, despite warnings from residents, contributed to and likely caused 79 people to be dead or missing. This was a policy failure that led to avoidable deaths and, says McKee, "it is impossible to achieve a comprehensive understanding of events like Grenfell Tower without confronting the political determinants of health and challenging the forces that shape them." The inequality and vulnerabilities of the poor are echoed by many of us. Bochen Cao and colleagues (doi: 10.1136 / bmj.j2765) grouped countries according to the Human Development Index and examined the effect of variation in cancer mortality rates on longevity. Countries with the greatest resources benefited the most in life expectancy as a direct result of improved cancer mortality. A key message here, from a devastating fire in a London tower block to uneven global progress in longevity, is that health professionals have a responsibility to ensure that the weak are not silenced, ignored or discounted. We must, in McKee's words, with a nod to Virchow, give voice to the voiceless. The above published in a prestigious magazine of a developed country, if Virchow lived in Latin America or sub-Saharan Africa, what would he think? I do not know, what can be inferred, when he manifests the search for wealth, by large economic consortiums. As a pathologist, Virchow analyzes the situation and looks for the root cause. We must not forget that we are human beings, we belong to the same species. As the poet Salvador Diaz Mirón said, "let no one enjoy the superfluous, while someone lacks the strict", this was written 100 years ago, and inequality still persists, the indifference that hurts when a poor person has no voice, this is seen daily in our population, mainly in the indigenous, women and without economic resources. We can and must do something, and this is solidarity with all our brothers and sisters regardless of social status or skin color. For this, education is fundamental, especially at home, where we should To teach the principles and values that we Mexicans have had for centuries, but that have been lost. Let us physicians be the current that leads to the search for those principles and values that our parents and grandparents have inherited from us. One must be privileged, and that is honesty with ourselves and our fellow men. Let us give the best of ourselves, and this is achieved by continuous preparation in knowledge, skills and humanism. Not to be so is to be an unethical person, a bad person. Let us be the transmitter of those who have no voice.

TEACHER

Nothing nobler than the vocation of teaching. The teacher who in a give and take amalgamates with the student. Giving the best of himself, to form better women and men. How much dimension exists when the destiny is teaching, and this is perhaps the most complex and transcendent destiny, because to devote oneself to the difficult task of teaching requires enthusiasm, but above all, vocation. He who sacrifices himself for the good of others, who guides his students towards the conquest of knowledge through teaching that moves, the truth that excites, the energy that galvanizes, has to be a teacher of a great destiny, and thus with the strength of this passion for truth and freedom of man, moving great obstacles, to build day by day a lasting work, the work of the transformation of man, in the professional that society requires. Teaching is a task that requires a profound structure of knowledge and full conception of teaching; of knowledge, because it is the basis and foundation, of teaching, because it is motivation and dynamism. And, in this mixture, we understand that the student requires intellectual and physical freedom; to realize himself as a human being, it is evident then, the need to understand him, and thus, with the intensive force of judgment, to guess the pearl of intelligence that seemed to be hidden in the student's conscience here is where the teacher and his deep intuition, makes him give his life, where his individuality becomes plurality, where he lives for himself and for others and thus enter the colossal world of true teaching. This is precisely the difference between the mediocre teacher and the successful one, between the ordinary and the extraordinary, because positive results are the consequence of work, dedication, effort and motivation. It is important to know, but more important than knowing, is knowing what to do with what you know. Knowledge is a treasure that provides happiness to the extent that it is transmitted and that without the pleasure of communicating it, knowledge would mean nothing. The teacher's reason are the students, restless and indifferent, respectful and disrespectful, responsible and irresponsible, assistants and absentees, restless and serious. Those who transmit us their problems and their achievements, their encounters and misunderstandings, the complicated and the happy, those who protest about everything and those who question everything, and when they want to, they rival and challenge us. All this is part of the profile of these exceptional and beloved beings, called students. Students who today are the nodal part of the intellectual task. The teacher's permanent commitment is to continue questioning ignorance, to reproach indolence, to reject the superfluous, to turn each student into a new man and to achieve in him, transformation, evolution, change in the rhythm of his own history.

FEAR AND POVERTY IN THE PANDEMIC

The pandemic has highlighted how much we need each other and how important care is in our societies. Isolation has had a very violent impact on the most vulnerable people (elderly, dependent or chronically ill people) and mental health problems are worsening among citizens. The COVID-19 has taken more than 190,000 people in our country, most of them dying alone and unable to grieve in a natural way. In the pandemic, we are all afraid of dying, some more than others. In the face of fear, various social responses to COVID-19 are observed, among them denial, that is, some people do not believe that the virus exists or deny the risks, others accept it; there are two ways of accepting the risks or falling into panic. The uneasiness and fear is present in older adults because it has been found that they are more likely to be victims of COVID-19. However, all ages are at risk. Young people do not follow health recommendations, whether at parties or at the beach. And, with cynicism they cynically refer that they have to live their lives, regardless of the lives of others, an unacceptable selfishness. This affects the population, mainly the social groups that are at a disadvantage and have a greater risk of falling ill and dying, since due to the characteristics of their environment they are more exposed to risk factors and at the same time have fewer protective factors or resources to face illnesses. Social inequality is a characteristic of Mexican society. INEGI reports 50% of poor people. That is why pandemic mitigation measures such as frequent hand washing, use of mouth coverings, healthy distance, staying at home. And, the vaccine is a hope to get out of this difficult situation. Fear of contracting COVID-19, the consequences of the pandemic are not affecting everyone equally. The most vulnerable sectors suffer a double impact in terms of health and psychological consequences. But also social, economic, cultural and environmental consequences that affect them more profoundly. It combines a series of new ethical conflicts with structural problems related to inequality and poverty. It is known that the gap is not only economic, but also inequality in the exercise of human rights, the capacity for autonomy, and the recognition of social groups. It is well known that the gaps do not only refer to the economic or means dimension, but also include inequality in the exercise of autonomy and recognition, particularly for some social groups. Everyone can recognize that injustice reigns around them and must therefore be an enthusiastic supporter of helping those who have less. A woman alone cannot take on the world. A man alone dies alone, thinking that he has no common destiny beyond shared misery. And this does not have to be so. We have too little time on the planet to live in fear. Fear and poverty are the consequences of the pandemic.

WOMAN SOURCE OF INSPIRATION

To Lupita Arroyo, my inspiration

Every woman is a sacred story, a value in itself. There is no love more sublime than a woman when she is a mother, a grandmother, a wife, a companion.

Human beings would not exist without the presence of women. She is the one who gives life, in her organism is formed that new being, which is the future of humanity.

The woman is a prodigy, a marvel of nature, an example of this is when her blood is transformed into milk, few such wonderful events exist.

A woman should be loved, respected and cared for, it is not understandable that a man abuses a woman. With verbal or physical violence, there is nothing more cowardly.

It has been said that if a human being is born in Mexico, and three conditions are met: female, indigenous, poor, his or her destiny will be adverse. So we must all avoid this situation.

March 8th, a day to celebrate women, or rather to vindicate their presence. On this day let us make a reflection, to remember the years of struggle through the years. Since ancient times women have been considered inferior, and although it may seem untrue, in many countries this is a reality.

Let us honor women, who despite the existing machismo, non-valuation, discrimination, have fought for equality and justice, in a long way that still does not end. Since prejudices are still observed only 'for being a woman.

Let us give thanks to woman, without her, life would have no meaning. Blessed is he who finds his destiny in a woman, and greater happiness if she accompanies him.

Woman is the perfection of the universe. God created her to make mankind happy. Life cannot be understood without her. That is why this March 8, if you are fortunate enough to have a mother, grandmother, wife, daughter, partner, tell her how much you love her, and respect her.

NON-MALEFICENCE

PRIMUM NON NOCERE

"First do no harm". This principle obliges us to avoid physical or emotional damage and harm in the application of procedures or interventions. We must avoid doing harm, it is an ethical duty, for all of us who dedicate ourselves to medicine. It is not simply a matter of doing the right thing, because that is how we consider it according to our principles or values, but we must guarantee that the result of our actions is beneficial; there is a supreme good, which is the patient's wellbeing. In clinical medicine, causing iatrogenesis, due to lack of knowledge, by not providing adequate treatment. The principle of non-maleficence together with that of beneficence and justice, in addition to respect and dignity, are made manifest in the Belmont Report, which reports the study of Tuskegee in the United States of America, in 1972, in which the course of latent syphilis is followed in more than 400 African-American people, these people were not given specific treatment, although antibiotics had already been discovered for more than 30 years. Or in a clinical laboratory without validated quality control, a false result value can be reported and cause harm. Hence the importance of laboratory personnel being constantly updated and professional. The patient does not know whether a laboratory meets quality control requirements, whether the flow cytometer is properly calibrated for CD4/CD8 lymphocyte count, and the antiretroviral therapy he or she will receive depends on that result. There is no excuse for not controlling quality, since we will cause harm, as was proscribed more than 2000 years ago by Hippocrates of Cos. If we take care of patients, let us be congruent, let us perform the functions for which we are prepared. Do no harm or harmlessness. This principle obliges us to avoid physical or emotional damage and harm in the application of procedures or interventions. Since the time of Hippocrates, more than 2,000 years ago, the physician has been considered to have a power, the power of healing. However, over the years, that power has sometimes been degraded. As reported in January 2016, a renowned physician sexually assaulted a black female patient, (1) in one of the most prestigious academic hospitals in the USA. It happened right in the emergency room, a place she went to in hopes of receiving care, and initially no one believed her. When semen analysis showed that, in fact, she was right, that this doctor had drugged her and proceeded to ejaculate on her, many questioned how this could have been possible. To most health care personnel, this would seem surprising and hard to believe. Probably his power, prestige and sense of invincibility were all factors that really made him feel he could get away with it, how many similar cases are known. There are doctors who are considered non plus ultra, cases of sexual, physical and psychological abuse are reported (2) and most of the time nothing happens. If we say we are ethical, let us be so.

1. One night at Mount Sinai, Aja Newman went to the emergency room for shoulder pain. Her doctor was a superstar. What is the worst that could happen? The Cut, Oct 15, 2019.

2. Fnais N, Soobiah C, Hong Chen M, Lillie E, Perrier L, Tashkhandi M et al. Harassment and discrimination in Medical training: a systematic review and meta-analysis. Acad Med. 2014; 89 (5): 817-827. doi: 10..1097.

PANDEMIC, A LESSON FOR HUMANITY

It is in these times of pandemic where we live situations that will probably affect us on a daily basis, and that will change our way of living, is the contingency caused by the coronavirus (SARS-CoV-2), first identified in the city Wuhan, in China, in December 2019, the disease caused by SARS- COV-2, which quickly evolved into a global pandemic that spread first in Europe, then in the United States and finally in Latin America, causing the collapse of health systems, mainly due to lack of ventilators, personal protective equipment, beds in intensive care units and personnel trained in critical care medicine. Arriving in Mexico in February of this year. Therefore, prevention measures such as healthy distance, use of mouth covers, frequent hand washing, staying at home, to mitigate the spread was the goal of saving lives. Currently with the presence of the pandemic SARS VOC-2, which has caused so much havoc in the population in December 2020 more than 100,000 deaths in our country. A Pandemic that was not expected and that the world was not prepared for. In recent Mexico there were epidemics of Spanish flu, cholera, influenza, but nothing compared to the current pandemic. Therefore, health systems must be transformed and initiatives must be promoted to help overcome exclusion, inequity and barriers to access and timely use of comprehensive health services, which is a task for all those involved in the health sector. It has been 40 years since the declaration of Alma Ata that declared "health for all in the year 2000", and no progress has been made in combating inequity in health care, and various mechanisms have been accentuated, such as the segmentation and fragmentation of health systems. This has caused people to receive medical attention depending on their place of work or their ability to pay out of pocket, causing those with more resources to have access to better services. In addition, there is a multiplicity of medical infrastructure, which has led to the centralization of the treatment of ailments, instead of attending to the individual's health in a comprehensive manner. It is in these times of pandemic where the human being needs the human being. Where the health team must have maximum security measures. Not having this means leaving everyone defenseless. Governmental authorities, as well as the population must be aware, co-responsible, and comply with sanitary measures. It is everyone's task. This pandemic leaves us with questions such as: Will we learn to take care of our health and that of all? Will we have the opportunity to learn in an ethical sense? What is the value of agreeing to a recommendation of what should or should not be done to take care of life if we are not capable of recognizing the other? These and other The questions that this pandemic has left us with, the promotion of instances that allow us to strengthen the recognition of others is surely not an easy path, and we will have to find ways to do it. This is the lesson that this pandemic leaves us. Let us be the good ancestors of our descendants.

RECOMMENDATIONS FOR FATHER'S DAY

Son as a man, you know that in your 40s, some "retirement planning" needs to be done. And I don't just mean protecting your finances. There's something more important: protecting your health. Good health is essential to doing everything you want to do in the coming years and decades. Deteriorating health can set in and darken a man's future. But you can keep yours bright! According to these recommendations:

1.- Mediterranean diet. This diet is the most recommended, remember to avoid red meat (once a month), limit alcohol intake (a glass of red wine a day), remember that alcohol is degraded in the body by an enzyme alcohol dehydrogenase, found in the liver, this exists in limited quantities, when exhausted, acetaldehyde is formed, which causes liver damage, mainly cirrhosis. Eat fish, legumes and mainly green vegetables, eating nopales for example in salad is a great idea. Say no to sugar and sweeteners, it is a proven risk for diabetes. So you should take care of your weight, having a scale in the bathroom is a good practice, since you can weigh yourself day by day, and thus control your weight. Drinking two liters of water a day, in this weather will help us not to dehydrate, this contributes to a better mood.

Exercise 30 minutes a day, if you can swim better, sometimes work, idleness, prevents us from exercising, as you know the best exercise is swimming, if you can not practice it walk steadily and vigorously, at least 30 minutes a day, it is desirable to strengthen the muscles, for this if you can go to the gym, great. Sometimes this is not possible due to multiple factors, so having in the bathroom a pair of dumbbells of 2 kilograms, is a good measure, we can exercise, accompanied by push-ups and squats, 10 at least.

3.- Stress Control, as you know it cannot be avoided, it is a biochemical reaction, but it can be controlled by means of exercises, such as, if you are in a state of stress, squeeze your toes as much as possible, with this most of the hormones such as adrenaline, go to the feet and not to the heart, breathe deeply and take the air out slowly. Do not give more importance to things than they have. Do not make assumptions, most of the time they are unfounded, act on real data.

Smile, try to be in a good mood, try to make others happy, by doing so you are also happy. You can be happy, it all depends on you. Happiness means to be fun and cheerful. It means not taking yourself as seriously as you do. to lose the joy of living. Happiness as joy is very closely aligned with the feeling .that I call abundance, because I feel that joy arises from the belief that you have the things you think you need to be happy, that your life is already abundant in a certain way. Happiness as a feeling of serenity. Serenity has to do with a sense of calm and tranquility. Happiness as a sense of interest. Interest has to do with being attached to something, to an object, or person, or activity. It is closely related to curiosity. That is, you can think of curiosity and interest as two sides of the same coin. Finally, happiness can be associated with fun. We all know that happy people laugh easily at themselves. It is true that laughter increases happiness levels.

5.- Realize yourself, first as a human being, be generous, it is proven that he who gives, receives more, especially with those who have less, always give the best of you in your profession, update yourself, remember that the patient does not know how good you are in your profession. Always give more. If you can travel, get to know other cultures and people, it will bring you joy and peace. Take care of your family, when you have your children, teach them the good way, be an example for them. Tell them every moment how much you love them and that you are proud of them. Take care of your wife, because she is the companion of your life and the one who will take care of you when the years go by and your children are gone, she will be your ally in your loneliness. Always keep in touch with your sister and nephews and nieces. Don't forget your parents, especially your mother. Honor them, so that you may have long life (according to the Bible). Be sincere, always speak the truth. And thank God for being here, with all those who love you.

REFLECTION TO A STUDENT

The dedication at work, the kindness of gratitude, kindness, the transcendence of friendship, the verticality of honesty, when these virtues are integrated into the willpower, the result is success. Give yourself at work, give a plus, an extra, always, this will make you stand out from everyone else, especially when you start a new job, a new position, your boss will have a good impression of you, continue with this commitment to always give a little more, so when for some reason, you can not do your job. Your boss will consider you, and will say that it is something occasional. The goodness of gratitude, nothing more appreciated by everyone than to be grateful, first with God, with life, with all those with whom you relate from the garbage man, to the most important people with whom you have to share, saying "thank you", ennobles you. The pleasant kindness, be kind, as your parents taught you in early childhood, being kind does not cost anything, especially with the female sex, take care of women, especially yours, those of your family, at work, in society. Remember if you go in a transport where there is a woman standing or an elderly person, give them the place, help them to go down a staircase, always with a smile on your lips. The transcendence of friendship, nothing more important than having friends, but friends are like flowers if you do not water them, that friendship ends. You have to cultivate friends, talk to them, greet them, and accept them as they are, we are all different. Those friends who do not give you their friendship unselfishly, just put them aside from your life. The verticality of honesty, being honest, in these times where it seems to be a thing of the past. Be honest first with yourself, with your family, at work, with society. Remember, have what you get with honesty, so that you can be a worthy person, and your children, full of pride, can say, my father was an honest person, it is true that he does not have much money, but he is a worthy person. What you get, always do it honestly, do not worship the golden calf, do not get carried away by the false prophets, where they tell you that wealth is easy to acquire, distrust them. Be true to yourself. Do not give up, not even when you are defeated, remember Alma Fuerte when he says: "Do not feel like a slave, not even when you are a slave; trembling with fear, think yourself brave, and attack fiercely, already badly wounded. Have the tenacity of the moldy nail that, now old and dull, becomes a nail again; not the cowardly stupidity of the turkey". Be a man of profit, integrity, loyalty. Remember Vincent Lombardi, American soccer coach of the Green Bays with whom he won two Super Bowls, among his phrases that you surely know is "Winning is not everything, but wanting to win". There is only one place in my game and that is first place" "We didn't lose the game, we ran out of time".

RESPECT IN MEDICINE

The word **respect** comes from the Latin word respectus and means **"attention"** or **"consideration", according** to the dictionary of the Royal Spanish Academy. Respect begins in the individual, in the recognition of the individual as a unique entity that needs to understand the other. It consists of knowing how to value the interests and needs of another individual. This principle is based on respect for the autonomy of the individual, which is essentially based on respect for people's capacity for self-determination in relation to certain individual choices. Respect for dignity is of paramount importance. Article 51 of the General Health Law establishes that the patient or user has the right to obtain timely health services of suitable quality and to receive professionally and ethically responsible care, as well as respectful and dignified treatment from technical and auxiliary professionals. The right to respect is sometimes violated. Therefore, it is necessary to start with ourselves, to respect ourselves, our family, our work, our co-workers, the Institution we belong to, it is a requirement that we must fulfill. Knowing our own value and honoring the value of others is the true way to earn respect. Respect is exercised when we show appreciation and care for the value of our fellow men. Respect is not in intelligence, but in love for others, it serves as a guide and inspiration to care for and honor them. If there is respect, there must be trust, "A trust in the face of a conscience". In medicine, trust in front of a conscience is fundamental, patients come to the doctor because they trust him. To be trusted is the priority, if it is not so only the conscience will make it known. For this reason, scientific knowledge is primordial, it must be continuously evaluated, this is the only way to achieve continuous improvement, to be ethical, with the values that we all appreciate such as respect, honesty, reliability, in a pleasant environment where daily work is performed, leaving behind the search for power and money as an end. That is why we must strive to promote and make known the good to do, especially in young people, to forge awareness in them. In the conviction that they not only have a professional duty towards the patient, but also an intimate duty towards themselves. To be ethical, respectful, reliable, responsible. To follow the rules that are followed in a group or a community, such as keeping silent in certain circumstances or respecting the areas and services created for others or disabled people. Respecting others is about recognizing their importance as people who inhabit the world and share life with you, about knowing that each of them is your neighbor, your fellow human being. The list includes your family members, your teachers and friends, your neighbors, but also anyone you pass on the street, even if you don't know them. Learn to be kind and affectionate with your environment: do not throw garbage in the street, respect children, the elderly, men and women, the differently abled, plants, pets, the environment. Build little by little the world where you want to live. Respect is the recognition of the inherent value of oneself, we must have faith in our own being, with integrity and integrity, to respect ourselves, this is the essence of our being.

UNIVERSAL HEALTH

Health care systems in different countries have evolved over time, with some countries offering private insurance including ours, other universal health care or a mix between the two. In most high-income, mainly European countries, health care is considered a human right and is provided universally, usually free at the point of care. The United States has developed a fractured for-profit system that is substantially more expensive than its European counterparts and offers poorer outcomes than health care systems in other high-income countries, while leaving a substantial proportion of Americans without health coverage. And, in Mexico? there is a fragmented health system, different health institutions, public and private health care. In an attempt to unify health services, towards a universal health system, the policy of "universal health coverage for everyone everywhere" was established where quality medical care and humanism must be received. That is why since 2001 in our country, public policies were developed to bridge the gap in health care, to provide health coverage and protect the population against catastrophic expenses derived from it, and thus promote the constitutional mandate of the right to health protection for all Mexicans, which in the paragraph added to Article 4 stipulates: "Everyone has the right to health protection". However, the right to health is not the same as the right to health protection. It is appropriate to point out that the former is broader, while the latter seems to refer, rather, to the obligation of the State to develop positive actions aimed precisely at protecting health or repairing it when it has been affected. No one should have to choose between good health and other vital needs. In an attempt to make health care universal for all Mexicans, what was called "Seguro Popular" was created. Its purpose was to provide protection to the non-eligible population through public and voluntary health insurance, aimed at reducing out-of-pocket medical expenses and promoting timely health care. With the new government of the Republic, the "Seguro Popular" was terminated and the "Instituto Nacional de Salud para el Bienestar" was created. The main objective is for the population to live healthier, to get sick less, to receive adequate care when they do get sick, to avoid premature death and to improve their quality of life. For health services to be truly universal, it is necessary to move from health systems conceived around diseases and institutions to health systems conceived around and for people. So that "Health for all" becomes a reality and not just a wish.

BEING A DOCTOR IN THE PANDEMIC

I feel alone in the hospital, 30% of the staff left for union leave due to comorbidities, 5% leave without pay, scheduled vacations, and those infected with SARS-CoV2, finally 50%. These are the words of a physician who is seeing patients. Feeling lonely, he recalls his entrance to the Faculty, why did he study medicine? He remembers "I like to help people", "to do good to others", "to take care of the sick". An experienced doctor tells him that studying medicine is a career of sacrifices, that the parties are over, there is no time for girlfriends. That by the time they finish their studies, most of their classmates will already be married, with families and established. On the other hand, the doctor will settle down around the age of 30; he will not enjoy watching his children grow up; he will not be at home every night, because his duty calls him, whether it is to be on duty at the hospital or to take care of the sick who require it. And, currently in the face of the SARS-CoV2 pandemic, his life is at risk. After the interview with the aspiring physician, his response is invariable: "It doesn't matter, I want to study medicine, because I want to help". Remembering Dr. Ignacio Chávez

(1) which in its ideology tells us, "it is advisable that whoever starts a career in medicine, obtains in reality a student's registration for a course that does not end. Slaves of a duty that conscience imposes and that everyone claims. And no freedom takes away more liberties, nor impedes more rest, nor detracts more from the legitimate expansions of the body and spirit than that which everyone demands and no one grants, no one thinks of the rights of the doctor-man and everyone demands the abnegation of the doctor-priest". It is in this pandemic that the physician will find himself before an implacable judge, his conscience, impossible to evade, not even when he has tried to avoid all risk with guilty abstentions. His duty is to protect the patient. But what happens if he is afraid of getting sick or infecting his family, if he does not have the appropriate personal safety equipment, and he has all the responsibilities and feels his commitment to the patient, he is obliged to do so. This is where assertive medicine, lex artis, Hippocratic principles such as "first do no harm", ethical principles and moral values should prevail in the physician. The patient expects the physician to be an anchor, a bridge between patient, disease and family. On occasions, the patient feels desolate due to the disease, such as Sars2 Covid-19 infection, and when the last breath of life arrives, he cannot say goodbye to his loved ones. According to Antonio Corral Castanedo (2), the patient finds himself on an island, with minimal contact with his family, due to the bureaucracy that prevails in some health systems. When the patient enters the hospital, he is subjected to machines and apparatuses that do not give him any explanation, between analyses and X-rays, examinations that he does not know what they are for and what they are looking for, that stun him and about which nobody explains anything, in the midst of which he hears very little. breath, few words; he is lost. It is there where the doctor, like a lighthouse, points out the light to the patient, since he longs for someone to look at him, to analyze his state of mind, his shocks, his fears, his loneliness. The

sick person, physically and, consequently, psychically mutilated, disturbed and diminished, looks for a handle; he looks for someone to help him bear and share the anguish engendered by the disease; someone to cure his specific ailment, his own. The doctor, like a lifeline, must speak a kind word, console the patient, his family, and many times give fatal news to a family that spends hours in the waiting room, without knowing anything, anguished over the fate of their loved one. The sick person wishes to be diagnosed and treated, to be helped through the streets of ailments, the necessary formalities, the days of hospitalization. That the doctor may hold tightly that childish hand, that childish existence, in which the life of any sick person becomes, no matter how adult and experienced he or she may be. Thus the sick person in the midst of the pandemic, the soul of the sick man, who seeks health, who requests above all a warm help, a comfort, a clarification, for his ills, his ailment that, although they are physical, affect his spirit, sometimes he still feels tragically and painfully ignored and abandoned, knowing that he will no longer see his loved ones in these difficult days due to the SARS-CoV2 pandemic. The physician asks God as did the Jewish physician Maimonides who only desires knowledge, to help his fellow man. The physician will accompany the sick person, will be his guide, his messenger, interpreter, a support, in the midst of all those who struggle to cure him, to consider him in his totality, to know his complexity, his personality, to successfully reach the recovery of his existential destiny. And, that the doctor and the patient do not feel alone, as if they were on an island in the midst of desolation. Coming to the conclusion that conventional success is not real success, not even for conventional reasons. Success is having served and done good.

References

1. Chávez, Ignacio. Ideario. Colegio Nacional, 1997.

2. Corral Castanedo, Antonio. Praise and nostalgia of the family doctor. Commemorative Year of the 250th anniversary of the foundation of the Royal Academy of Medicine and Surgery of Valladolid. 1981.

SOLIDARITY

A group of medical and nursing personnel from the State of Campeche were transferred to Mexico City to support the care of patients with COVID-19 in different medical units of that entity. This is to speak of solidarity, understood as the social expression of human fraternity in all fields of coexistence and which is an essential condition for the integral development of people and the edification of the future of humanity. What is desirable is not the same as what is possible, but Campeche shows solidarity in these difficult days of the pandemic. Solidarity is a fundamental human value at all times and even more so now. In these days of the COVID-19 pandemic, solidarity translates into actions that make people act for the benefit of health. For example, if the majority of a population is vaccinated against certain diseases, this will benefit all the children in that community, or if the quality of air, water and food is controlled, people with asthma, diabetes or obesity will improve their health. If we consider solidarity as a collective commitment that acts in favor of health. Let us not forget that we must be in solidarity with each other, by taking care and taking sanitary measures in the face of this pandemic, such as keeping a healthy distance, using mouth covers, washing our hands frequently, and staying at home. All these solidarity measures should be a norm in the population, so that the ravages of the pandemic do not affect us as much as in other places, this is the responsibility of each one of us. Solidarity is a sign of empathy towards those who are going through a difficult situation, understood as a moral feeling that allows us to put ourselves in the place of the other, that is, put ourselves in their shoes. Solidarity is sometimes not given its value, due to the influence of the concept of quality of life based on individuality, where everyone is concerned about their own welfare, regardless of the other. On this occasion Campeche gives an example of solidarity. It is not enough to be in solidarity in the midst of the vicissitudes and difficulties of everyday life, it is necessary to recognize the importance of dignity, to recognize each and every one for what they serve and contribute. Solidarity, always closer to the person, can easily reach where justice does not reach, either because of human incompetence or its limitations, and through affection, understanding and love, corrects abuses and lack of justice. To be in solidarity not only with the care of the human body, but also with its feelings, its soul, its spirit, everything that makes up the human being as a whole. In these difficult days of the pandemic, solidarity is the adhesion or unconditional support to causes or interests of others, especially in compromising situations such as the current ones.

ARE VITAMINS USEFUL?

Vitamins are heterogeneous compounds essential for life, which when ingested in a balanced way and in essential doses promote the correct physiological functioning. Since childhood we have always had a relationship with vitamins, currently in medical practice in childhood vitamins such as A and D are recommended, and then vitamins are still recommended in adulthood, mainly vitamin B for fatigue, improve work performance, and in old age vitamins are still recommended, to have an old age with fullness of faculties, this mainly by the media, mainly television. It is important to consider that the sale of vitamins in the United States, in 2010, represented 28 billion dollars, probably in Mexico, a considerable amount is also used. Representing a great business for pharmaceutical companies, perhaps much of this money would be used in other benefits to have better health conditions. That is why two articles and an editorial published in the journal Annals of Medicine Interne in 2013 are relevant, in the first one a multicenter, double-blind, randomized, placebo-controlled study, where 1700 subjects over 50 years of age were studied, all of them had presented a myocardial infarction, previously one group took multivitamins and the other placebo for three years. The results showed that vitamins did not protect the heart. In the second study, to know the effect of vitamins and cognition, 600 male physicians aged 65 years and older were studied, who were administered multivitamins for 12 years, and their cognitive abilities were evaluated. As a result, the vitamins did not stop cognitive decline. Also the USPSTF reported 26 studies on the pros and cons of vitamin supplements to prevent heart disease, cancer and overall mortality. As a result, insufficient evidence was found for the benefit of vitamins. In the Editorial, it refers to stop spending money, since a well-nourished adult does not need vitamins, as there is no clear benefit and it does comment that high doses of vitamins such as beta carotene, vitamin E and vitamin A, can be harmful. Beta carotene has been associated with increased risk of lung cancer in smokers and vitamin E supplements with overall mortality. With its exceptions, such as vitamin D, in patients with this deficiency, research should continue to be carried out since there is no solid evidence of its benefit.There is a group that does need vitamins and these are pregnant women, where folic acid is of great importance to prevent neural tube defects in newborns and in people who have vitamin deficiencies, such as pellagra, scurvy, beriberi, when a lack of folic acid is detected.of vitamins and not only for commercial reasons. Ingesting vitamins is necessary for the body, since it can synthesize them, but these can be acquired in sufficient form in fruits and vegetables, a good example of this is the Mediterranean diet. The consumption of vitamins should be judicious and with scientific knowledge, otherwise we will only be spending money and with possible damage. Let's try to have a balanced diet, avoid processed foods, sugar, walk every day, we all want to be healthy, and when we end this life, death will find us enjoying full health.

DREAM

Not sleeping well? There are factors that prevent you from falling asleep, such as fear of getting sick, problems at work, family relationships, economic problems, or drinking coffee after mid-afternoon, among other reasons that can make you lose sleep. Sleeping is an essential activity for life that, for thousands of years, has aroused great interest due to the difficulty of understanding its meaning, purpose and for being surrounded by a certain mystery because of its similarity to a situation of passing death. In fact, in Greek mythology sleep is represented by the winged god Hypnos, twin of Thanatos, god of non-violent death, both being sons of the goddess of the night, Nyx. Similarly, in our sayings we find equations between one and the other: "sleep and death, brothers they seem", since, apparently, in both there is a functional paralysis, temporary in one case and definitive in the other. Nothing could be further from the truth: sleep is an active process at the physiological and brain activity level. If we do not sleep well, we may feel fatigued and fatigue is a symptom, not a disease, and different people experience it differently.Fatigue caused by stress or lack of sleep usually disappears after a good night's rest, while other fatigue is more persistent and can be debilitating even after a good night's sleep. Scientists divide sleep into two main types: REM (rapid eye movement) or dream sleep, and non-REM or restful sleep. Surprisingly, they are as different from each other as each is from waking, but both can be important for energy.Non-REM sleep consists of three stages. Sleep specialists believe that the last of these, known as deep sleep or slow-wave sleep, is the main time when your body renews and repairs itself. This stage of sleep appears to play the most important role in energy, improving your ability to produce ATP, the body's energy molecule. In deep sleep, blood flow is less directed to the brain, which cools considerably. At the beginning of this stage, the pituitary gland releases a pulse of growth hormone that stimulates tissue growth and muscle repair. Researchers have also detected an increase in blood levels of substances that activate your immune system, raising the possibility that deep sleep helps prepare the body to defend against infections and slow aging.

Therefore, it has been recommended:

1. It is necessary to create a suitable environment to be able to rest and to not interrupt sleep during the night, because environmental conditions will greatly affect the moment of sleep. rest and the ability to fall asleep. To make the most of your rest during the night, you need to sleep on a comfortable mattress, with a suitable pillow, and in a room where you feel comfortable. When it is time to fall asleep, it is advisable to have little light, little noise and a pleasant temperature. It is highly recommended to have the TV off. In addition, you should use the bed only for sleeping. What do I mean by that? Well, the bed should not be used for other things, for example, to play console games, to work on the computer or to eat.

2. Follow a sleep ritual

If you have trouble sleeping, you can try having a bedtime ritual. For example, take a warm bath with some music to relax you and then have a herbal tea before going to bed. It is also important to be relaxed at bedtime.

3. Watch your diet

Food can influence our sleep, as both what and when we eat can affect our overall well-being and can be a problem when it's time to go to bed. A balanced diet will always be beneficial for our organism, but it is also important to keep a schedule for meals. Dinner should not be heavy, but neither should we go to bed hungry because it can cause us to wake up during the night in search of food.

4. Do not take stimulants after mid-afternoon.

Coffee consumption is widespread in our culture, but caffeine stimulates the brain and interferes with sleep. Consuming it in the morning may be a good option, but coffee, tea or cola should not be consumed after mid-afternoon, especially if you are sensitive to its effects.

5. Exercise

Regular exercise helps people sleep better. Its beneficial effects, however, depend on the time of day the exercise is performed and the individual's general physical condition. Some experts warn that exercise performed in the morning does not affect nighttime sleep, and even helps people sleep better, but if it is performed very close to bedtime and the exercise intensity is high, it is likely to cause sleep disturbances.

6. Diet

Many studies seem to indicate that sleeping after eating brings many health and mental benefits. Therefore, taking a nap will have a beneficial effect on your well-being and can increase your alertness, your concentration, your productivity, and will improve your memory and learning ability. A nap of no more than 30 minutes.

7. Alcohol

Do not drink alcohol before going to sleep, because although it will help you fall asleep faster due to its depressive effect, it will alter the subsequent sleep phases and cause you to wake up during the night, preventing you from getting the necessary rest and reducing the quality of your sleep.

8. If you can't get to sleep, get up.

If you are ever unable to fall asleep, get up and engage in a sleep-inducing activity, such as a relaxation technique or reading a book. It is better not to stay in bed, as this will increase your anxiety as time goes by.

9. Always go to bed and get up at the same time.

Having a schedule for going to sleep and waking up will allow your body to start the processes that will trigger sleep in advance, and help you to optimize your internal clock and, therefore, the quality of your sleep.

10. Clear your head

Stress, worries or discomfort from something that has happened during the day can interrupt your sleep. If this happens to you, you should take some time away from bed for self-reflection, as this can help you figure out what's going on with you and what you need to do to fix it. If you can't stop worrying and feel like you've lost control, you need to learn to manage your thoughts.
So let's try to sleep better!

Bibliography

• Ferrie JE, Kumari M, Salo P, Singh-Manoux A, Kivimäki M. Sleep epidemiology-a rapidly growing field. Int J Epidemiol 2011; 40(6):1431-1437.
• Freeman, D. et. al. (2017). The effects of improving sleep on mental health (OASIS): a randomised controlled trial with mediation analysis. Lancet Psychiatry, 4(10): pp. 749 - 758.
• Merino, M. et al. (2016). Healthy sleep: evidence and guidelines for action. Official document of the Spanish Sleep Society, 63(2).
• Taheri, S., Lin, L., Austin, D., Young, T., & Mignot, E. (2004). Short sleep duration is associated with reduced leptin, elevated ghrelin, and increased body mass index. PLoS medicine, 1(3), e62.

ARE YOU GOING TO A PARTY?

In the midst of the coronavirus pandemic, Campeche is in green light, thanks to the participation of the population that has followed the recommendations of the health authorities. You are probably tired of following the health recommendations, staying at home, keeping a healthy distance, not attending parties, gatherings with family and friends, and have thought about getting tested for the virus causing the pandemic, which is SARS-CoV2, a type 2 coronavirus, the cause of severe acute respiratory syndrome. Waiting for it to come out negative to go to a meeting, to a party to have fun, without keeping a healthy distance, not using mouth covers, not washing your hands because, according to you, it came out negative. This is very dangerous. It has been reported that groups of young people are tested for COVID-19 on Thursday with the hope that it will come out negative on Saturday, so they can attend their meeting. This may cause a false sense of security, which could mean that the meeting could become a site of infection for a highly contagious virus. The result you got on Saturday morning was from Thursday when you tested and it said negative, it says nothing if it is still negative on Saturday. If a person tests shortly after becoming infected, but before the virus has reproduced enough copies of itself, a test may not detect the virus and give a false negative result. It can also happen that a person may be exposed to the virus right after testing on Thursday and be contagious on Saturday. Remember that people can be infected with COVID-19 and not show symptoms of illness. So we need to emphasize, use of mouth coverings, healthy distance, hand washing, staying home. We have to focus on reducing transmission. Follow public health recommendations. This is the only way we will be able to stay in green light and get out of these difficult days of the pandemic, which has caused so much pain. We are the ones responsible for this to end. And, even when the vaccine is available, we must not lower our guard and continue to take care of ourselves for the good of all.

A PROPOSAL, LET'S LIVE LONGER.

If we want to live well, if we choose to live well, we can have significant reductions in the risk of developing diseases. It is all up to us and no one else. We all fear death to a greater or lesser degree. Death in old age is of course inevitable, but death in mid-life is avoidable. Although the only sure thing in the universe is death, that is why we must take action to avoid death by disease in mid-life. There are numerous studies on how to live healthier, there are training programs, messages on television, where we are invited to eat less salt, reduce the intake of red meat, watch our body weight, do not smoke, reduce or avoid the intake of alcoholic beverages, or also diets such as the Mediterranean diet. In reality there is little adherence to these recommendations, why are they not followed and if they are followed it is minimal, an example is exercise, 30 minutes a day is recommended, either walking or some other sport, and it is not done, because it is more comfortable to be sitting watching television, and the human being always looks for comfort. It is said to avoid excessive intake of calories, but it is not done, since we are accustomed since early childhood to cola soft drinks, junk food, that although we know they are harmful to health, we continue to ingest them; it is so little will that we have, that government agencies restrict their sale in schools, or increase taxes for consumption. The increase in caloric intake favors the presence of obesity and diabetes, which as we know is one of the main causes of morbidity and mortality. Not to mention red meat, which, due to its high content of saturated fats, is harmful to health. One aspect of great importance is salt, it is recommended to limit its use, but it is present in all foods such as sausages, seasonings, fried foods, snacks, bread, so we must be careful and read labels to control salt intake. Although smoking has decreased, it is still present and is observed in the young population, so at this stage of life we must be aware of the danger it represents. Six actions to achieve a good life:

1. Regular exercise
2. No smoking
3. Maintain a low body mass index
4. Vegetable-based diet
5. Limiting alcohol consumption
6. Taking care of salt consumption

If one practices 5 of the 6 actions, compared to people who do none, it was found that:

➢ A 67% reduction of the risk of cardiovascular disease

➢ Reduction of type 2 diabetes incidence by 73%.

➢ Decrease in cancer development of 20-25%.

➢ 65% reduction in dementia

➢ And the decrease in overall mortality of 32%.

What should we do, spread the actions, the rewards are real, let us be an example for the family of each one of us, let us form disciples, who in cascade spread the actions. Through persuasion, training, dissemination, we will avoid early deaths. And when we reach old age, let it be of fullness, independent, enjoying life, let us be like good wine, which when it ages becomes cognac and not vinegar. But for this we must comply with the actions that have been proposed.

ANTI-COVID-19 VACCINE, A LIGHT AT THE END OF THE TUNNEL

Severe acute respiratory syndrome coronavirus 2 (SARS-CoV-2) infection and resulting coronavirus disease 2019 (Covid-19) has affected tens of millions of people in a global pandemic. Safe and effective vaccines are urgently needed as the Covid-19 epidemic continues to grow. In some parts of the country, hospitals are reported to be overcrowded with patients and their families. There is currently one hope and that is the vaccine, but even with it, the return to normality will depend more and more on the success of mitigation measures such as healthy distance, frequent hand washing, use of mouth covers and staying at home whenever possible. However, there is currently high transmission of the virus, which puts great pressure on hospitals, intensive care units and health care workers. There is concern about the growing perception that with vaccines the pandemic is over and it is not. Scientists welcome the first convincing evidence that a vaccine can prevent COVID-19, but questions remain about how much protection it offers, to whom and for how long. The vaccine to be used was licensed by COFEPRIS, and is based on genetic instructions known as messenger RNA (mRNA), which prompts cells to produce a SARS-CoV- 2 protein that trains the immune system to recognize the virus. We know that vaccines have benefited humanity because they allow the immunization of people from any age, making them the most successful and cost-effective intervention in health. According to the World Health Organization, every year three million deaths are prevented in the world and the disability of 750,000 children is avoided. In spite of this, approximately two million children per year die from preventable diseases, which represents approximately 25% of all deaths of children under five years of age, hence the importance of immunization. The prevention of a given disease represents a fundamental fact for public health, since it is better to prevent a disease than to treat it. However, there are people who argue that they should not be vaccinated, that their autonomy, their decision, should be respected. Without forgetting that public health should prevail over private health. This has caused great havoc in the health of the population due to people who do not want to be vaccinated, such is the case of measles, a disease that was practically eradicated, is reappearing. Article 144 of the General Health Law states that vaccination against communicable diseases, preventable by this means of immunization, as determined by the Ministry of Health, will be mandatory under the terms established by said agency and in accordance with the provisions of this Law. What seems to be a step forward for vaccination holds the promise of saving countless lives and a pathway out of what has been a global disaster. It is uncertain how long the vaccine will last to protect against COVID-19, so it is imperative that we continue to take care of ourselves.

VACCINATION

Is it ethical not to vaccinate children? The reason for this question is that in recent years communicable diseases such as measles have appeared in the United States and in some European countries. Parents refuse to vaccinate their children, fearing that the vaccine will cause autism. There is no link between vaccines and autism. There is no scientific evidence linking the MMR vaccine (measles, mumps and rubella) with autism or autistic disorders. This unfortunate rumor was born from a single 1998 study linking the measles vaccine to autism, but the study was soon found to be seriously flawed, after which it was withdrawn by the journal that published it. Although vaccine-preventable diseases have become rare in many countries, the infectious agents that cause them continue to circulate in others. In today's interconnected world, they can easily cross geographical borders and infect anyone who is not protected. For example, measles outbreaks have occurred in unvaccinated populations in Austria, Belgium, Bulgaria, Bulgaria, Denmark, France, Germany, Greece, Italy, the Russian Federation, Serbia, Spain, Switzerland, Tajikistan, the United Kingdom, the United States of America and the Russian Federation. The vaccines are safe, rigorously tested throughout the different phases of clinical trials, and continue to be regularly evaluated after they are marketed. It is much easier to suffer serious injury from a vaccine-preventable disease than from a vaccine. For example, polio can cause paralysis; measles, encephalitis and blindness. Some vaccine-preventable diseases can even be fatal. The benefits of vaccination far outweigh the risks, and without vaccines there would be many more cases of illness and death. Vaccines induce an immune response similar to that produced by natural infection, but unlike natural infection, they do not carry serious risks of death or disability. Being vaccinated is always the best option, even if you believe there is a low risk of infection. Deadly diseases that seem to have passed through all but the eradication stage reappear when immunization rates drop, as seen in recent measles outbreaks in the United States and Europe. If the population is not vaccinated, infectious diseases that have become infrequent could reappear. In Mexico, polio, diphtheria, measles and neonatal tetanus have been eradicated thanks to the commitment of the population and the health team. Let us not allow these diseases to return. Let's vaccinate children. To stop vaccinating children is unethical, immoral. They depend on us. Let us not let them down.

VEJEZ

Why do we age? You have probably wondered why one person ages faster than another. The probable answer is genetics. It has been proven that when parents are long-lived, there is a great probability that their children will reach advanced ages. In addition, advances in medicine and environmental conditions. In the last century the average age at which an individual lived was 60 years, currently it is estimated that women live 78 years and men 74, these are only statistics, since there are people who reach 100 years of age and those who do not live past 20. Are we programmed to live a certain number of years, is a question that has been asked for many years. Oscar Wilde in his book The Portrait of Dorian Grey, sells his soul to the devil in order to stay young, or Aldous Huxley in his work Brave New World, where the human being when he reaches 30 years old, stays with that physiognomy, does not age, does not get sick, but when he reaches 80 years old, he must end his current life. The human being does not want to age, that is why there are a lot of cosmetic products used by men and women to delay aging, spending large amounts of money for this purpose. It is known that the more you eat, the faster you age and this is because when food is ingested it oxidizes, when it oxidizes it originates free radicals that shorten the telomeres, which protect the DNA of the cell, and this makes the cell can no longer divide originating what we know as wrinkles, which is why taking care of the weight is to avoid premature aging. When we go to a reunion of high school classmates, after 40 years, we meet with classmates and we realize that not all have aged equally. It has its explanation it has been pointed out that a person can have what has been called ageotype and these can be four, metabolic, immune, hepatic and nephrotic, a person can have one or a combination. People have a genotype which is the genetic information and a phenotype which can be observed as a physical characteristic, eye color, they also have an "ageotype" which is a combination of molecular and other changes that are specific to a physiological system. These changes can be measured when the individual is healthy and relatively young, such as in the metabolic ageotype taking care of the amount of glucose, creatinine in the nephrotic ageotype, liver enzymes in the hepatic ageotype, erythrocyte sedimentation rate in the immune ageotype, just to mention a few. To reach old age is an achievement, but we must reach it in the best health conditions, for this we must take care of our health since childhood, have a healthy diet, avoid tobacco and alcohol control, practice exercise thirty minutes a day, do meditation such as yoga. If we understand this we will probably be able to have a healthy old age. So that when we reach the end of our days we will be in good health.

TRUE GENDER EQUALITY

March 8 marks International Women's Day, established by the United Nations (UN) in 1975. This day commemorates the struggle of women and the constant search for gender equity. So it is necessary to empower women, as it has been proven time and time again that empowering women has a multiplier effect and helps promote economic growth and development in the world. There is nothing more beautiful than women. Women are the most important support for human beings. Since she takes care of him from birth, she feeds him with breast milk which is a prodigy of nature, the woman's proteins through prolactin are converted into milk and this is the fundamental food in the development, as it contains all the nutrients necessary for proper growth. In addition, it contains defenses (antibodies) that protect the baby against infections and contributes to strengthen the mother-child bond, favoring an adequate psychomotor development. When the human being grows, the mother takes care of him, feeds him and watches over him. Without the woman, life cannot be explained. Sometimes women do not receive the same treatment, an injustice that has been present for centuries. In our culture there has been an unfounded machismo, considering women as inferior beings. Violence against women cannot exist, it is cowardice. When it occurs, it must be punished with full rigor, as in the case of rape. What happens in this heinous crime, the rapist pays a fine and spends an average of 5 to 10 years in prison, and if he is influential sometimes has no punishment. Meanwhile the woman's life is destroyed forever. Meanwhile, when the rapist gets out of prison, he returns to cause the damage. That is why some voices have requested that the rapist be castrated. But if justice is dispensed by men with a misunderstood machismo, little can be done. Our grandfathers used to say that a woman should not even be touched with the petal of a rose. It has been said that the worst thing that can happen to a human being born in Mexico is to be a woman, poor and indigenous. We must all fight against this injustice that has no place in today's Mexico. They are our mother, sister, daughter, granddaughter, all of them women. Ending all forms of discrimination against women is not only a basic human right, it is also crucial to promote the social development of humanity. Women's empowerment is a necessary and indispensable prerequisite for achieving true gender equality. Let us take care of women, they are our most valuable treasure, without them humanity has no future. Not only on this International Women's Day should they be recognized, but every day, an equal treatment, a fair salary, a thank you for ever.

VIEJISM

Old, five letters, some people consider it an insult, and look for euphemisms such as full-grown adults, older adults, senior citizens. When it is a stage of life, such as childhood, adolescence, adult and old age. However, there is a prejudice in society against the elderly. It has been called old age prejudice, stereotypes, discrimination, isolation, marginalization, mistreatment and lack of respect. It is based on the belief that, in old age, people are less attractive, capable, intelligent, and productive. Aging is a stage of life, related to older age, a natural and gradual process, continuous change, irreversible and integral (biopsychosocial). Health problems occur in the elderly, which deteriorate the quality of their lives, affect their autonomy, are costly and lead to old age. In Campeche, life expectancy has changed from 50 to 6 years at the beginning of the 20th century, and in the 21st century, from 70 to 80 years. In itself, the increase in life expectancy is an indicator of the success achieved by individuals, society and its institutions in the search for wellbeing and development. The human being does not want to age, that is why there are a lot of cosmetic products used by men and women to delay aging, spending large amounts of money for this purpose. Do not resist to grow old, many are denied the privilege. What should be done to care for the elderly? Privilege their dignity, access to health services in a timely and effective manner, as well as culture, education, personal care throughout life. Old age must be empowered. Planning for aging is everyone's duty. No to overprotection and abandonment. Yes to dignity. The human brain can produce new neurons until the age of 90 (Nature Medicine, March 15, 2019). Michelangelo Bounarroti, 89 years old, Winston Churchill, 91 years old, Pablo Picasso, 92 years old and many more. Never mind being old, never mind glasses, never mind gray hair, never mind life, and living it with zest. It doesn't matter to be slow and with wrinkled skin, it matters what has been lived and the struggle won. It doesn't matter the bent back, it doesn't matter the life and honey harvested. It does not matter the time that passes and goes. Life matters at any age. María Cecilia Popelka.

HIV/AIDS, THE OTHER PANDEMIC

According to the World Health Organization, in 2019, 690 000 people died from causes related to the human immunodeficiency virus (HIV), and 1.7 million people were infected. In Campeche to date, more than 4,000 people have been reported. These overwhelming figures underscore the fact that much remains to be done, such as developing a safe and effective HIV vaccine, while antiretrovirals with improved efficacy and duration continue to be developed. Thus, it is imperative to provide treatment rapidly to individuals so that sustained viral suppression can be achieved, prevent at-risk individuals from acquiring HIV infection, rapidly detect and respond to emerging clusters of infection, eliminate HIV infections and deaths, as well as HIV-related stigma and discrimination. The implementation of educational actions through different strategies such as sexual behavior with the use of condoms, elimination of multiple partners and the consequent maintenance of a stable partner. Educational activities also have a valuable value for the de-stigmatization and de-stigmatization of those affected by the disease in question. HIV/AIDS patients, for example, have not only exposed the weaknesses of biology, psyche, culture and morals of the individual and postmodern society, questioning behaviors and values of various kinds, but have also tested the union and integrity of the affected patients' families. Homosexuals, bisexuals, drug addicts or so-called sex workers of both sexes should not be discriminated against, just because they are at greater risk of exposure to the virus and that, like any human being, the HIV/AIDS patient has the right to health protection, which should be provided with equity, accessibility, opportunity, effectiveness and high human quality. Recalling that fundamental rights cannot be promoted or exercised as long as they are not known. The full understanding that nothing is asked for by imploring compassion, but from the conviction that dignity is the source of the right to health, must emerge with vehemence. This is where rights emanate from, which is why favors are not asked for, rights are exercised.

VULNERABILITY BY COVID-19

China in December 2020, a coronavirus causes severe acute respiratory syndrome, as the causative agent (SARS-CoV-2). The World Health Organization (WHO) designated this new entity as coronavirus disease 2019 (COVID-19). After the first cases were reported, COVID-19 spread rapidly around the world; on March 11, WHO declared this new disease a global pandemic. In Mexico, the first imported cases were described on February 28, 2020, and local transmission was detected as of March 24. As of February 1, 1,869,000 infections and 159,100 deaths have been reported. Greatly affecting the economy in all productive, service and educational sectors. To mitigate the pandemic, measures such as healthy distance, use of mouth covers, staying at home, frequent hand washing have been recommended. However, the impact on the population infected by the coronavirus has been devastating. The presence of traffic lights in relation to the risk, cause desperation in some sectors of the population. And, when drastic measures are taken, a free society can only endure it for so long. There must be a way out of this catastrophe, easing restrictions, especially when the burden may outweigh the unproven, theoretical and at best marginal benefit. And, that way seems to be the vaccine. The one that has been designed to be administered first to health personnel in the first line of care to COVID 19, older adults and so on to the entire population. Not forgetting the low-income, indigenous people, who often bear the greatest burden during public health disasters and their aftermath. The COVID-19 pandemic has been no different. Vaccinating people who are deprived of their liberty, in psychiatric hospitals, people in street situations, ensuring compensation in case of an adverse effect to the vaccine is an ethical imperative. Mortality is much higher in areas of high poverty than in wealthier areas. Therefore, it will be of great importance to rapidly vaccinate members of low-income minority populations. The risks of sudden loss of income or access to social support have consequences that are difficult to estimate and are a challenge to identify all those who might become vulnerable. Therefore, the vaccine should not be used as a bargaining chip, which for privileges can be accessed by people who do not deserve to be vaccinated at the time. Nothing is more immoral than to take away a benefit from a person in need. Vaccination against COVID 19 provides a stress test that will help organizations prepare for other challenges ahead. Thus, in the midst of the COVID-19 pandemic, the vulnerable groups are not only the elderly, people with poor health and comorbidities, the homeless, or the homeless, but also people from a gradient of socioeconomic groups who may have difficulty making financially, mentally or physically facing the crisis. That is why we must all show solidarity.

ENOUGH, ENOUGH

Sometimes we say enough is enough of lies, unpunctuality, carelessness, irresponsibility, corruption, illegitimate profit, vile cunning. For this we must change, first of all ourselves. Nothing is more dishonorable than a lie, because a lie makes us lose confidence. Let us be punctual, we are given to say an hour and arrive an hour later, to be punctual is to be respectful of the other's time, if we say 4 o'clock in the afternoon, it is 4 o'clock in the afternoon, not 5 o'clock. Let us avoid idleness, sometimes we leave everything for the last moment, for example, payment of tenure, taxes, license plates, etc. Since we leave it for tomorrow, that is to say for later, we must do things today, not tomorrow. Irresponsibility is so frequent, we must be responsible, answer for our actions, do not blame others, be responsible with ourselves, our family, society, to have a country that we would like to have. Corruption, that nefarious scourge that has permeated society must end, phrases such as "he who does not compromise, does not advance" should not exist. The illegitimate medro as achieving positions by cronyism or compadrazgo, not by own merits is something that must be fought. It is in early childhood where civism, good manners and ethics should be instilled, since youth is our hope. If we want Mexico to change our beloved Mexico, let us change ourselves first. Let us be better women and men, let us be proud to say that we are Mexicans, this will only be achieved with the participation of all. Those who act dishonestly must be punished, impunity must not prevail. When we are born we are not corrupt, dishonest or liars, it is the environment that fosters it. Hence the importance of ethical and civic education. Let us remember the poet Ramón López Velarde, when in his poem Suave Patria, he says "Like the sota moza, Patria mía, on a metal floor, you live by day, by miracle, like the lottery. Fifty times is the same the bird drilled in the thread of the rosary, and it is happier than you, Patria suave. And, with so many situations that our country has had, Mexico continues to be the loving mother, waiting for the best of her children. Our Mexico, our Campeche, In all the acts we perform. Let's be loyal, let's avoid illegitimate medro, the vile cunning. Let us respect human rights. Let us love life. Let us not allow the lack of values to be our common denominator, let us be ethical. Let us be congruent, with ourselves, with society, being honest, responsible, integral, are values that we cannot renounce. Let us love Campeche dearly, this is our Campeche, the Campeche of our children, there is no other. Let us love it, this is the only way to make Campeche and Mexico so dear to us, what it has always been, a homeland of which we are proud, where we will live to the fullest.

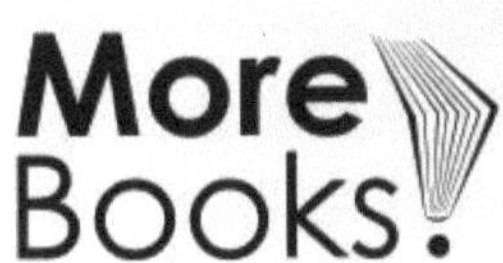

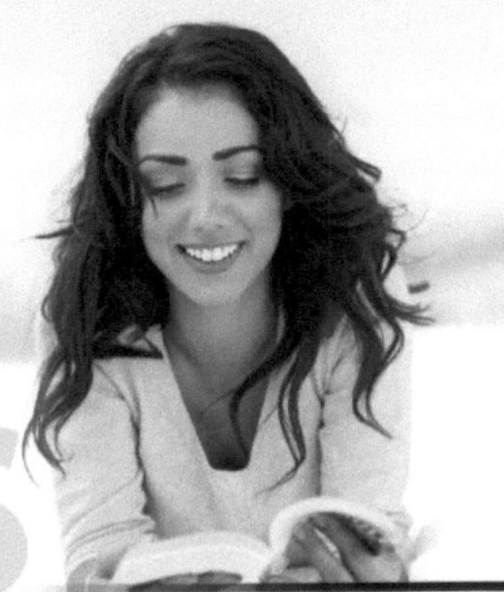

I want morebooks!

Buy your books fast and straightforward online - at one of world's fastest growing online book stores! Environmentally sound due to Print-on-Demand technologies.

Buy your books online at
www.morebooks.shop

Kaufen Sie Ihre Bücher schnell und unkompliziert online – auf einer der am schnellsten wachsenden Buchhandelsplattformen weltweit! Dank Print-On-Demand umwelt- und ressourcenschonend produzi ert.

Bücher schneller online kaufen
www.morebooks.shop

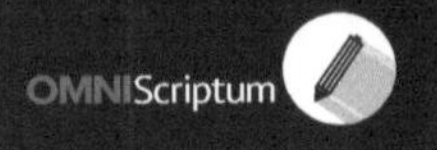